Amphetamines
and pH-shift Agents
for Brain Imaging

Amphetamines and pH-shift Agents for Brain Imaging

Basic Research and Clinical Results

Edited by
H. J. Biersack and C. Winkler

Walter de Gruyter
Berlin · New York 1986

Professor Dr. H. J. Biersack

Professor Dr. Dr. h. c. C. Winkler

Institut für klinische und
experimentelle Nuklearmedizin
der Universtität Bonn
Sigmund-Freud-Str. 25
D-5300 Bonn 1

This book contains 93 illustrations and 37 tables

CIP-Kurztitelaufnahme der Deutschen Bibliothek

Amphetamines and pH-shift agents for brain imaging : basic research and clin. results / ed. by H. J. Biersack and C. Winkler. – Berlin ; New York : de Gruyter, 1986.
ISBN 3-11-010772-4
NE: Biersack, Hans J. [Hrsg.]

Library of Congress Cataloging in Publication Data

Amphetamines and pH-shift agents for brain imaging.

Includes bibliographies and indexes.
1. Brain – – Diseases – – Diagnosis – – Congresses. 2. Brain – – Radiography – – Congresses. 3. Tomography, Emission – – Congresses. 4. Amphetamine – – Diagnostic use – – Congresses. 5. Amphetamine – – Derivatives – – Diagnostic use – – Congresses.
I. Biersack, H. J. II. Winkler, Cuno.
RC386.6.T65A47 1986 616.8'0757 86-6343
ISBN 0-89925-156-0 (U.S.)

 Typesetting and Printing: Buch- und Offsetdruckerei Wagner GmbH, Nördlingen. – Binding: Dieter Mikolai, Berlin. – Cover design: Rudolf Hübler. – Printed in Germany.

Preface

The development of ^{123}I-labeled amphetamine derivatives and their diagnostic application in connection with Single Photon Emission Computerized Tomography (SPECT) has opened up a new dimension for brain imaging in clinical practice during the last 5 years. Although since the mid-seventies Positron Emission Tomography (PET) has proved to be eminently suited for the clarification of questions concerning brain perfusion and metabolism, PET has remained restricted to relatively few research centers because of the extensive instrumentation necessary. In contrast, the widespread availability of radiopharmaceuticals labeled with single photon emitters, in conjunction with SPECT-systems, provides the possibility of their diagnostic use on a broad scale.

The experimental basis for the application of the new Single-Photon emitting tracers which show a high blood brain barrier permeability, has been established only relatively recently. For this reason it has only been possible for a few selected research groups to gain experience with these radiopharmaceuticals. The purpose of the symposium of the Rhineland-Westphalian Society of Nuclear Medicine, which was held in October 1984 in Bonn, was to bring together these groups in order to discuss both the experimental and the clinical data as far as currently available. The organizers were fortunate to be able to welcome most of the leading experts of the groups for an exhaustive exchange of ideas. The papers from the symposium are summarized in this book. The first part covers reports on basic research (preparation of labeled amphetamine derivatives, pharmacokinetics, and metabolism). Data are included on diamines and other potentially useful ^{123}I- or ^{201}Tl-labeled compounds and ^{99m}Tc-propylenaminoxime (PAO) derivatives. Two talks on instrumentation problems complete this chapter. The second part deals with clinical results of brain imaging with amphetamines in cerebrovascular diseases, epilepsy, migraine, and brain tumors. Problems of quantification of SPECT scintigrams and their clinical significance are also discussed.

Although it has been possible to gain additional experience with the new agents since the meeting in Bonn, the proceedings presented in this volume should be of fundamental interest both to radiopharmaceutical chemists and to physicians dealing with the diagnosis of brain lesions. If these proceedings can contribute to the wider use of SPECT for improved diagnostic results, than it will have fulfilled its purpose.

Bonn, February 1986 *H. J. Biersack and C. Winkler*

Contents

I Basic Research

II Clinical Results

I Basic Research

Pharmacology of Amphetamines

R. M. Baldwin, Tz-Hong Lin, Jiann-Long Wu, J. F. Lamb

Introduction

N-Isopropyl-p-iodoamphetamine hydrochloride labeled with ^{123}I (IMP, generic name iofetamine HCl ^{123}I) has received considerable attention since its original report for brain imaging [1]. However, relatively little is known about the precise fate of the molecule in vivo. This presentation will be divided into two parts: first, a brief review of the toxicology of IMP, and then a description of recent results on the metabolism of IMP in humans.

Toxicology of IMP [2]

The acute toxicity of N-isopropyl-p-iodoamphetamine hydrochloride was determined in rats, mice, and dogs (tab. 1). The intravenous LD-50 was found to be 46 mg/kg in rats and 82–94 mg/kg in mice. In dogs, no central nervous system effects were observed at doses up to 3 mg/kg. At doses of 10 mg/kg, some effects were seen, such as tongue thrusting and muscular contractions.

In subacute studies, rats were given 1.6 mg IMP per kg of body weight per day and dogs were given 0.1 mg per kg per day for two weeks. No physiological changes

Table 1 Toxicity of IMP

1. Acute toxicity: a) LD-50: 82 mg/kg in male and 94 mg/kg in female mice. 46 mg/kg in rats. b) No signs of central nervous system stimulation observed after up to 3 mg/kg doses in dogs. CNS effects were seen at 10 mg/kg.
2. Subacute toxicity: a) Rats: no significant treatment-related effect seen with doses of 1.6 mg/kg/day for two weeks. b) Dogs: no toxic or pharmacological effect seen with doses of 0.1 mg/kg/day.
3. Ames mutagenicity assay: not mutagenic.

were observed different from animals receiving a control dose of 0.9% sodium chloride solution.

The proposed human dose of IMP in routine clinical studies is 1.5 mg, or about 0.02 mg/kg for a typical patient. This is well below the threshold of pharmacological effect.

IMP was found to be non-mutagenic in the Ames test.

Pharmacokinetics

Based on the known metabolism of amphetamines [3, 4] four metabolites of IMP can be predicted (fig. 1): p-iodoamphetamine (PIA), resulting from dealkylation, p-iodophenylacetone (PIPA), resulting from deamination, p-iodobenzoic acid (PIB), resulting from further oxidation of the aliphatic side chain, and p-iodohippuric acid (PIH), the conjugate of p-iodobenzoic acid with glycine. Other metabolic paths, such as para hydroxylation, would not be expected for IMP because the para position is substituted with an iodine atom.

Early studies in rats demonstrated that the activity in brain consisted entirely of amines (IMP and p-iodoamphetamine) for up to 24 hours after intravenous administration [5]. The major metabolites detected in rats were p-iodobenzoic acid and p-iodohippuric acid; the major route of excretion was in the urine. p-Iodophenylacetone and iodide were detected in these experiments, but it wasn't clear if the iodide was endogenous or an artifact of the extraction procedures. p-Iodohippuric acid was identified as the major metabolite of IMP in humans as well [6]. Other studies have corroborated these findings [7, 8].

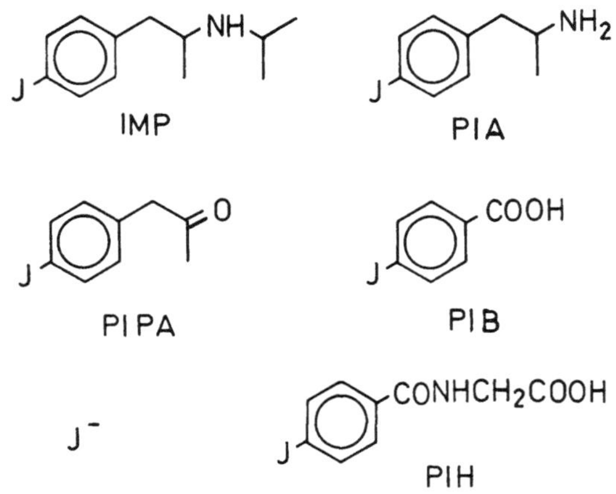

Fig. 1 Structure of IMP metabolites.

We recently carried out an analysis of the metabolites of IMP in normal human volunteers, completed only two weeks before this symposium. We haven't carried out detailed quantitative analysis of the data yet, so the results should be considered a preliminary report.

Seven subjects were each given 3 mCi ^{123}I IMP intravenously, and serial blood samples and urine were collected over a period of four days; each subject fasted for 5 hours before administration, and all received the same type of food about 6 hours after administration. This was intended to minimize variation in the pH of the urine, which is known to have a pronounced effect on the rate of excretion of amphetamines in the urine [3, 4]. The plasma was separated from the red blood cells and was then extracted with organic solvent. The organic extract was analysed by HPLC using an automated system assembled with a special sodium iodide scintillation crystal and digital interface to a microcomputer, which allowed detection of subnanocurie levels of metabolites. With gradient elution, baseline separation of all six suspected components (IMP, PIA, PIPA, PIB, PIH, and iodide) was achieved. However, in many of the biological samples, PIB and PIH were incompletely separated, and therefore these two components were counted together. The urine was also extracted and analyzed by HPLC.

The results are shown in the next series of slides. The total ^{123}I activity in the blood (fig. 2) showed an initial decrease to a minimum of about 0.9% of the injected dose in the blood pool at about 1–2 hours after administration, then increased gradually

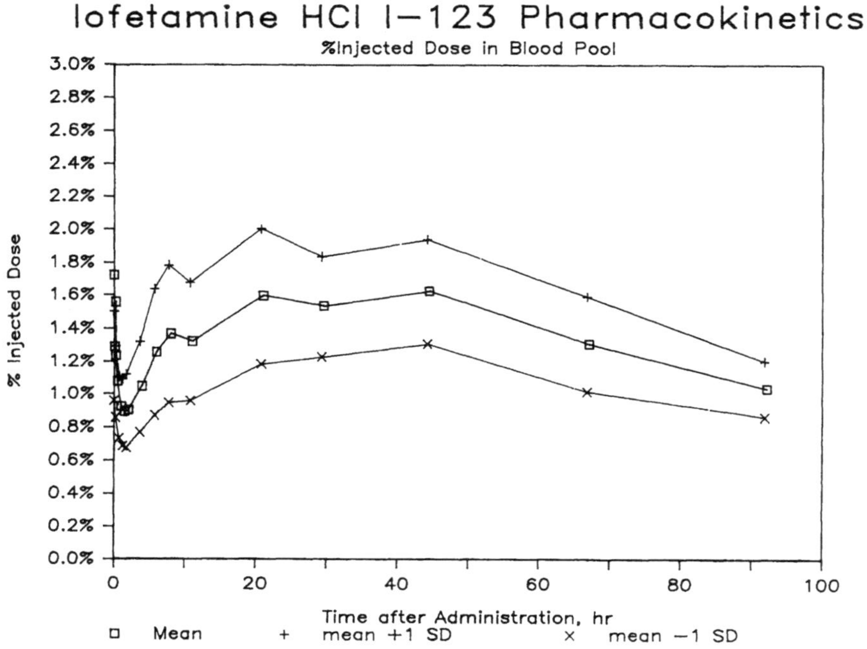

Fig. 2 % dose in blood pool.

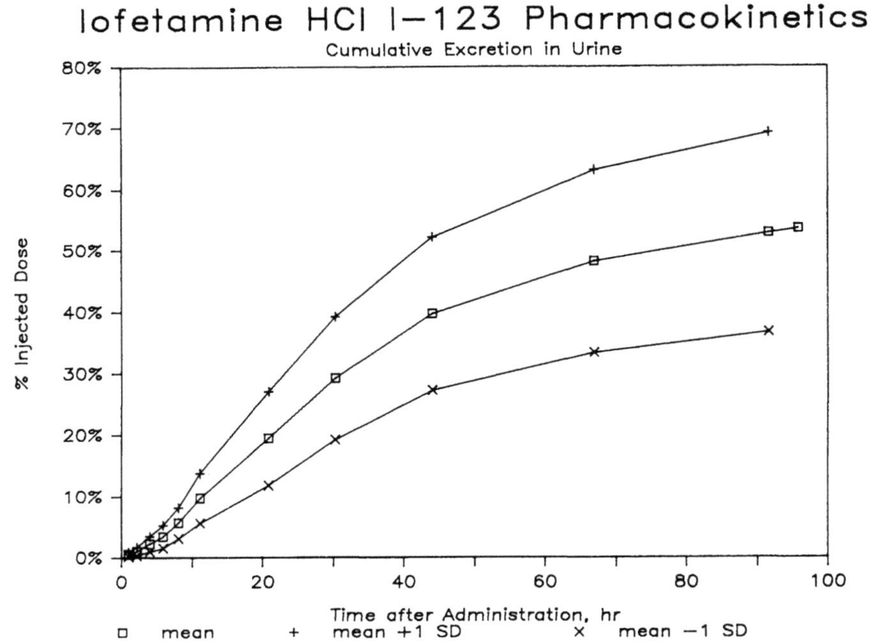

Fig. 3 % dose excreted in urine.

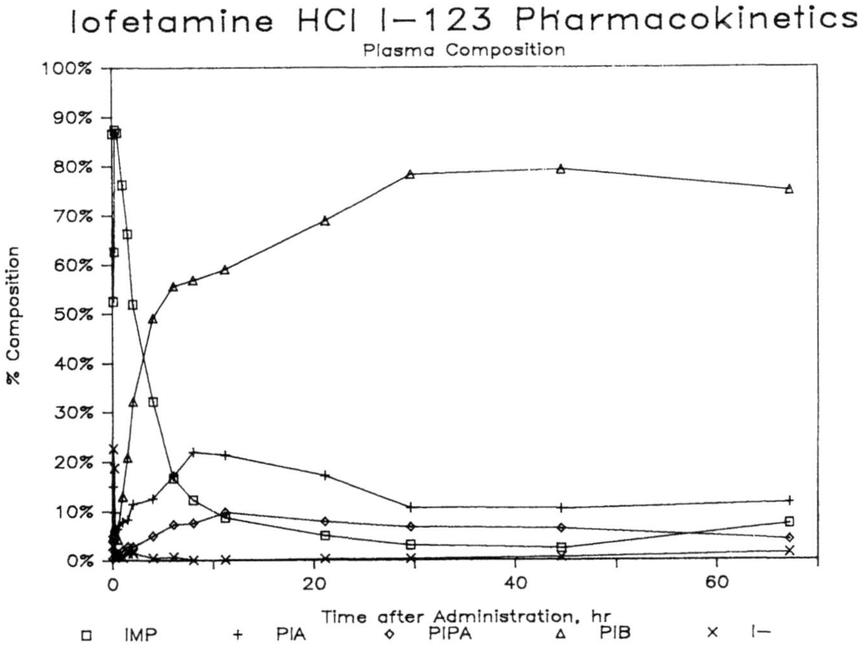

Fig. 4 Plasma composition after IMP administration.

to a peak of about 1.6% after two days, and then decreased again. The activity in the plasma followed a similar pattern. These results are consistent with previous studies [9, 10], which showed initial rapid clearance followed by a gradual increase on the first day; previous studies have not measured the activity beyond one day, however. The principal route of excretion was through the kidneys (fig. 3). On the average, about 20% of the injected dose was found in the urine after one day, 40% after two days, 48% after three days, and 54% after four days. The variability in the measurements of urinary activity was quite high after two days, probably because the subjects left the clinic after the second day, and complete urine collection was not achieved in every case. The total activity excreted in the urine after four days ranged from 31 to 75%.

If we now look at the composition of the plasma (fig. 4), IMP represented the major component immediately after administration (the first blood sample was taken 15 minutes after injection). PIA increased to a peak of about 22% of the plasma activity between 8 and 12 hours after administration. The major metabolite was p-iodobenzoic acid. The PIB content increased rapidly, so that it was the major component after about 8 hours, and continued to increase to a plateau value of about 75% of the plasma activity after 24 hours. PIPA, the ketone resulting from deamination, was present in only minor amounts, peaking at about 10% of the plasma activity between 12 and 22 hours. No significant levels of iodide were detected in the plasma. Because of radioactive decay and excretion of activity from

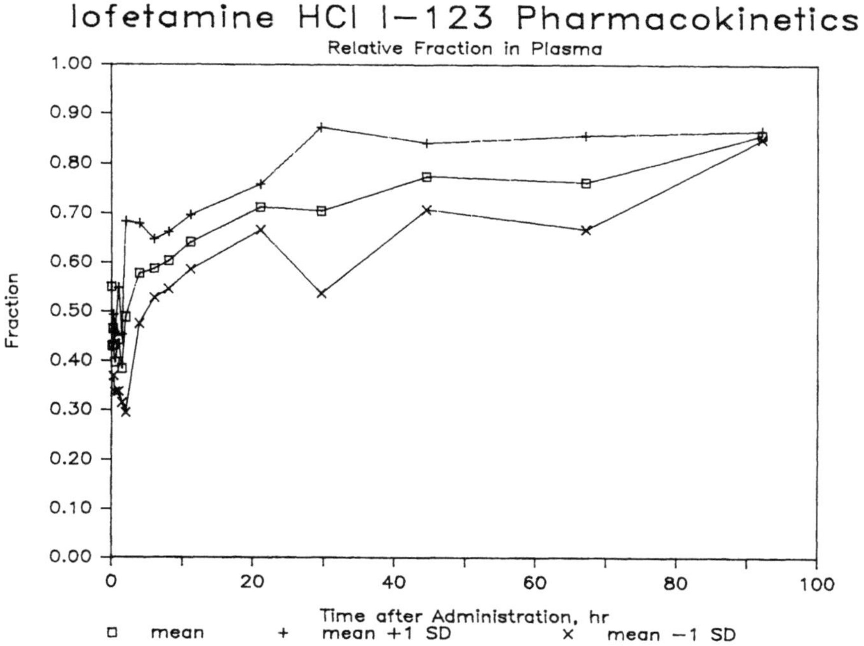

Fig. 5 Relative fraction in plasma.

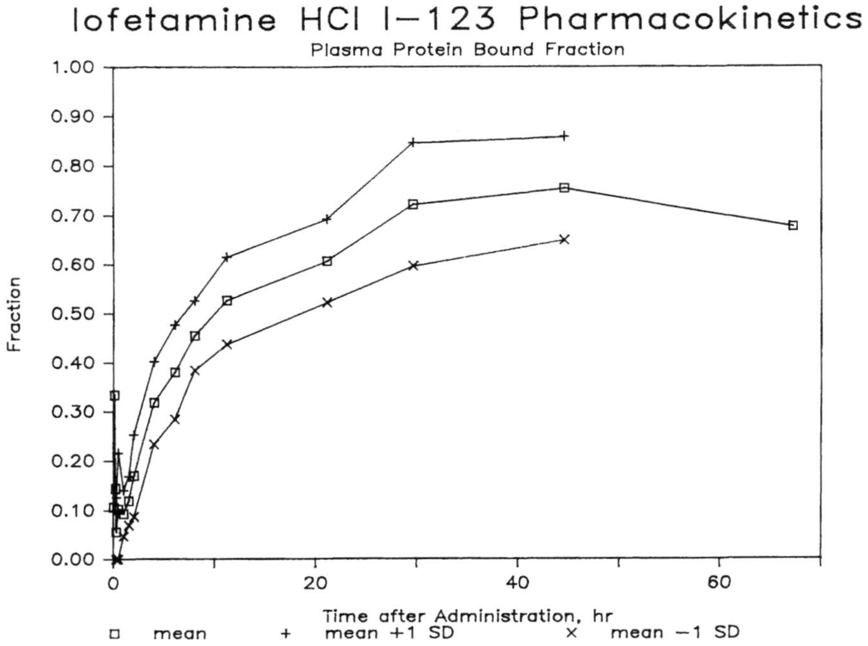

Fig. 6 Plasma protein-bound fraction.

the body, we were not able to analyze the plasma for metabolites beyond the second day.

The distribution of activity between the plasma and red blood cells increased from approximately equal distribution immediately after injection to about 80% of the activity associated with the plasma after 24 hours (fig. 5). The protein-bound fraction likewise increased from less than 10% bound immediately after injection to a plateau value of about 75% bound after 24 hours (fig. 6). This behavior parallels the increase in the proportion of PIB in the blood, and agrees with our experience that IMP is not bound by plasma proteins, but that benzoic acid is significantly protein bound, and with published results that IMP activity is freely exchangeable between red blood cells and plasma [6].

The composition of the urine reflected the plasma composition (fig. 7). From primarily amphetamines (IMP and PIA) in the first sample one hour after administration, the content of PIB (actually appearing as mostly PIH) increased rapidly to the dominant component within 8 hours after administration, with a plateau value of 60–70% of the urinary activity. PIPA was a minor component, peaking about 12 hours after administration. The content of PIA remained at a residual level of about 20% of the urinary activity up to the end of the experiment. In the urine, we did see significant amounts of radio-iodide appearing in the first sample and decreasing rapidly to background levels within 12–24 hours after administration. The quantity of radioiodide excreted in the urine could be accounted for from the

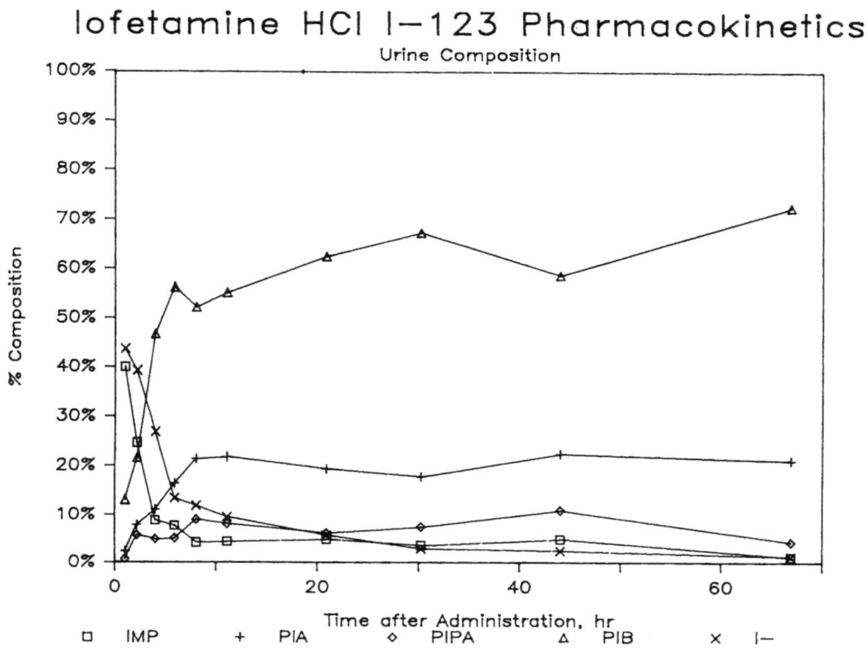

Fig. 7 Urine composition after IMP administration.

amount of iodide present in the injection solution (about 2–3%); together with the pattern of excretion, it is probable that the urinary iodide activity did not result from in vivo metabolism.

Our results suggest that there are multiple paths of metabolism, possibly reflecting the different organs in which the transformation takes place. From animal studies we know that the liver is the major source of polar metabolites, whereas the brain and the lung activity remains as mostly amines. In addition to the sequential degradation of the side chain of IMP suggsted by figure 1 (IMP – PIA – PIPA – PIB – PIH) there may be pathways that lead directly to the metabolites without the release of intermediates into the general circulation. Additional experiments will be necessar to explain the biochemical pathways more clearly.

References

[1] Winchell, H. S., R. M. Baldwin, T. H. Lin: Development of ^{123}I labeled amines for brain studies: localization of ^{123}I-iodophenylalkyl amines in rat brain. J. Nucl. Med. **21** (1980) 940–946.

[2] Lin, T. H., R. M. Baldwin, J. L. Wu: Development of ^{123}I-N-isopropyl-p-iodoamphetamine: Exploration, synthesis, and metabolism. 16th Japan. Conf. Rad. Radioisot, Tokyo, December 6.–8., 1983.

[3] Caldwell, J.: The metabolism of amphetamines and related stimulants in animals and man. In: Amphetamines and related stimulants: Chemical, biological, clinical, and sociological aspects. CRC Press, Boca Raton, FL, pp. 29–46, 1980.

[4] Lemberger, L., A. Rubin: Amphetamine. In: Physiologic Disposition of Drugs of Abuse. Spectrum Publishers, N. Y., pp. 31–63, 1976.
[5a] Wu, J. L., T. C. Bruggmann, T. H. Lin: Fate of ^{123}I-N-isopropyl-o-iodoamphetamine in the rat brain. 182nd Annual Meeting, American Chemical Society, N. Y., August 23.–28., 1981.
[5b] Wu, J. L., T. C. Bruggman, D. D. True et al.: Tissue distribution and metabolism of N-isopropyl-p-iodoamphetamine in rat. 2nd Int. Symp. Radiopharmacol., p. 97. Chicago, September 8.–12., 1981.
[6] Kuhl, D. E., J. R. Barrio, S.-C. Huang et al.: Quantifying local cerebral blood flow by N-isopropyl-p-[^{123}I]-iodoamphetamine (IMP) tomography. J. Nucl. Med. **23** (1982) 196–203.
[7] Rapin, J. R., D. Duterte, M. Le Poncin-Lafitte et al.: Chemical and pharmacologic aspects of brain cell tracers. Annales de Radiologie **26** (1983) 48–52.
[8] Rapin, J. R., M. Le Poncin-Lafitte, D. Duterte et al.: Radiopharmacologic studies of isopropyl iodoamphetamine. In: Functional Radionuclide Imaging of the Brain (Magistretti P. L. Ed.). Raven Press, N. Y., pp. 209–216, 1983.
[9] Delaloye, B., A. Bischof-Delaloye: Biodistribution of ^{123}I-Amphetamine: First experience and possible clinical applications. In: ^{123}I-Amphetamine (Perfusamine^{TM}). Proceedings of a Colloqium on diagnostic applications of ^{123}I-Amphetamine (von Schulthess, G. K., Bekier, A., Schubiger, P. A., Eds.). pp. 106–118. Wurenlingen, Switzerland, October 28, 1983.
[10] Bischof-Delaloye, A., J. P. Hungerbuhler, F. Regli et al.: Biodistribution of ^{123}I-iodoamphetamine in man. J. Nucl. Med. **25** (1984) 108.

Labelling of Amphetamines with ^{123}I

H.-J. Machulla, E. J. Knust

Introduction

Radionuclides which can be produced by means of a cyclotron are very well suited for labelling organic substrates which are to be applied in nuclearmedical diagnosis. Among these cyclotron produced radionuclides ^{123}I has particular advantages:

1. The half-life of 13.2 hours is short, on the other hand it is long enough to permit commerical distribution.

2. ^{123}I does not emit β^--particles which increase the radiation dose without contributing to the nuclear medical measurement, most important, however, is the emission of the γ-radiation with an energy of 159 keV in 80% of all decay events; thus ^{123}I is optimal for measurements by γ-cameras and single-photon-emission-tomographs.

3. Since halogens can be bound directly to carbon atoms, ^{123}I can easily be introduced into an organic compound and it is possible to take advantage of the nuclear-physical properties of ^{123}I in case of labelled metabolically relevant compounds. Metals such as ^{99m}Tc, on the other hand, need the introduction of chelating groups to perform binding to the molecule. Thus the polar and steric properties are drastically altered, resulting in a very different physiological behaviour of the compound when compared to the original substrate.

It has often been stated that radioiodinated compounds cannot be used in metabolic studies since they do not generally belong to the naturally occurring substrates. The successful application of radioiodinated amines and fatty acids, however, illustrate that compounds labelled with radioiodine can really be metabolic analogues. As we recently pointed out [1] new developments of radiopharmaceuticals labelled with ^{123}I will be promising if the size of the iodine atom, which is similar to the methyl group, is taken into account and when a radiopharmaceutical concept is established for a radioiodinated substrate. In the previous radiopharmaceutical studies it was observed that after introduction of an iodine atom alterations of the molecular polarity are so small that the lipophilic properties, which can strongly influence the physiological behaviour, remain practically unchanged.

Production of ^{123}I

A large variety of nuclear reactions are known for the production of ^{123}I and were comprehensively discussed by Weinreich [2]. Due to the cross sections, two reactions only have been used depending on the energy of the cyclotron available for the production. At high energy machines with proton energies between 65 MeV and 75 MeV, the radionuclide is produced via the $^{127}I(p,5n)$ $^{123}Xe(EC,\beta^+)$ ^{123}I process. The only important radionuclidic impurity is caused by ^{125}I ($T_{1/2}$ = 60 d) which can be kept below 0.2% at the end of production. ^{123}I commercially offered, occasionally contained more than this percentage of ^{125}I-impurity and care is advisable concerning the additional radiation dose applied to the patient.

At cyclotrons with proton energies below 40 MeV ^{123}I is obtained by proton irradiation of 96% enriched ^{124}Te via the $^{124}Te(p,2n)$ ^{123}I reaction. The important impurity ($\geqq$ 0.9% at the end of bombardment) is ^{124}I ($T_{1/2}$ = 4.2 d) which is produced by the $^{124}Te(p,n)^{124}I$ process, competing particularly at lower energies. Due to the emission of γ-rays with high energies (511 keV, 603 keV, 723 keV), the ^{124}I-impurity of 3% or more seriously decreases the quality of the scintigrams. Reichmann et al. [3] discussed the influence of the ^{124}I-impurity and showed that the effect on the image quality was underestimated. In case of brain measurements by single-photon-emission-tomography (SPECT) the background can increase from 18% up to 33% and thus, artefacts may be caused by the reconstruction procedures used in SPECT.

In the past years great efforts were undertaken in finding efficient procedures for producing ^{123}I with a minimum of radionuclidic impurities. The cyclotron groups in Vancouver (Canada), Eindhoven (Netherlands) and Karlsruhe (FRG) started to produce highly pure ^{123}I via the $^{124}Xe(p,2n)$ $^{123}Cs(EC,\beta^+)$ $^{123}Xe(EC,\beta^+)$ ^{123}I process.

In contrast to the situation in 1976, when the first panel on ^{123}I was organized by Weinreich and coworkers [4], sufficient quantities of ^{123}I are now available both in Europe and North America. Although the introduction of radioiodinated fatty acids and amphetamines for diagnosis of metabolic alterations in the myocardium and the brain has been opening new areas in nuclear medicine, the wide-spread use of ^{123}I was limited so far by the number of ^{123}I labelled radiopharmaceuticals.

Radiopharmaceutical Concept

Due to the nuclearmedical technique of performing measurements by γ-cameras and SPECT, a radiopharmaceutical suitable for diagnosis of brain diseases has to meet certain conditions: i) After intravenous injection the compound must rapidly be extracted out of the blood, ii) the uptake of the radioactive compound in the organ of interest, i.e. the brain, should be high and, iii) particularly with respect to registration by means of SPECT, a retention of the accumulated labelled compound is needed, i.e. the alterations of the radioactivity in brain during the period of measurement have to be neglegible.

For applying radioiodinated amphetamine derivatives in nuclear medical diagnostic procedures, the radiopharmaceutical concept ist based on the fact that biogenic amines are able to cross the blood brain barrier. Baldwin and coworkers [5, 6] prepared and studied a large variety of radioiodinated biogenic amines. They found the para iodo-N-isopropylamphetamine (IMP) to be one of the best compounds meeting the conditions mentioned above. As Kuhl et al. [7] showed the IMP uptake in brain to correlate directly with the flow of labelled microspheres within the first five minutes, IMP has been assumed to be an indicator for measuring brain perfusion. Since Baldwin's group did not observe any carrier effect on the brain uptake, the role of specific binding sites were excluded and it was proposed that high-capacity, non-specific binding sites were responsible for the accumulation in the brain. Details of the pharmacology of amphetamine and its alkylated derivatives are discussed in Baldwins proceeding chapter of this book [8].

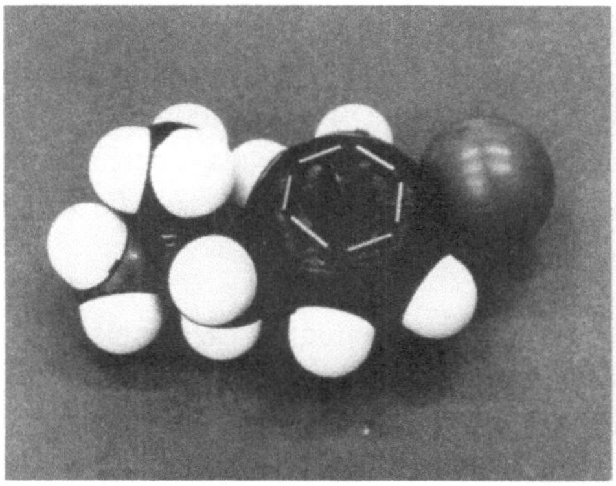

Fig. 1

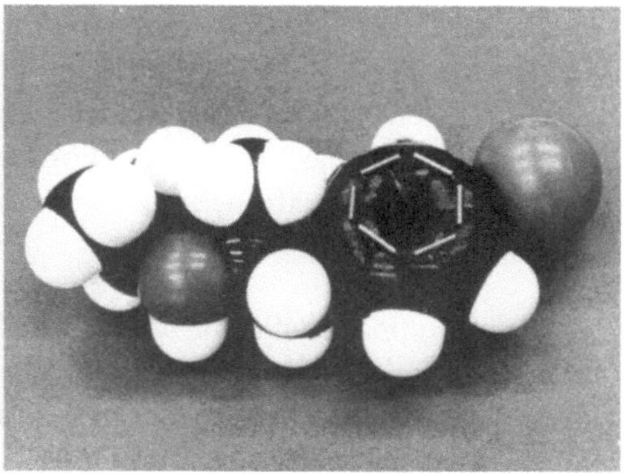

Fig. 2

Fig. 1 Molcecular model of p-iodo-amphetamine p-I-C_6H_4-CH_2-$CH(CH_3)$-NH_2.

Fig. 2 Molecular model of p-iodo-N-isopropylamphetamine p-I-C_6H_4-$CH_2CH(CH_3)$-NH-$CH(CH_3)_2$.

Figs. 1 and 2 show the molecular models of p-iodo-amphetamine and that of p-iodo-N-isopropylamphetamine. One clearly recognizes that the largely sized iodine atom, which does not effect the brain uptake if it is placed in the para position of the benzene ring. It is assumed that the nitrogen atom of the amphetamine is responsible for the interaction with the non-specific binding sites in the brain. The binding mechanism probably occurs via hydrogen bonding leading to a spatial separation of the aromatic ring from the N-binding region by two carbon atoms. Therefore, the iodine atom in the para position of the benzene ring does not decrease the brain uptake. If, on the other hand, the iodine atom is located in the ortho position, it causes sterical hindrance and lower brain accumulation is observed. N-alkylation by the isopropyl group, however, obviously does not decrease the brain uptake, evenmore it increases the lipophilicity and therefore was thought advantageous for accumulating in brain tissue.

Labelling methods

If radioiodinations are to be performed, methods should be chosen which allow the preparation with good radiochemical yields and with high specific acitivities. It often is discussed to carry out these reactions under carrier-free conditions, i. e. the labelled compound is obtained without any non-radioactive isotope product. This, however, is generally not possible since reagents always contain traces of halogens in the ppb to ppm range. The term "no carrier added", which was suggested as a better alternative, also is not useful because the reagents of different laboratories may contain different amounts of impurities and thus, different but unknown quantities of carrier are introduced into the reaction mixture. Therefore, the only clear approach is the determination of the specific activity of the product after the synthesis. The mass detectors used in the separations by highpressure liquid chromatography (HPLC) allow such an assay. If no mass is observed appearing simultaneously with the radioactive product peak, a limit of the specific activity can be calculated on the basis of the detection sensitivity of the particular mass detector. In this case the real specific activity may be considerably higher, but its lowest limit can clearly be defined.

Since the original studies of Baldwin and coworkers indicated no carrier effect on the brain uptake of IMP, the specific activity seems not to be of great importance. From the organic chemical point of view the amphetamine derivatives belong to the same group of aromatic compounds as the phenyl fatty acids, i. e. aromatic substrates which are clearly activated for electrophilic substitution reactions in ortho and para position. Therefore, the experiences in labelling phenyl fatty acids, as summarized by Machulla [9], could successfully be applied for the radioiodination of amphetamines. Since the electrophilic substitution yields in a mixture of two isomers, only the method of labelling by isotope exchange was taken into consideration, since it allows an iodination exclusively at one position of the ring. After Eisenhut [10] had shown the radioiodination of phenyl fatty acids by isotope exchange, the procedure was applied in a modified way in order to increase the specific activity by a factor of hundred. If the method is applied for labelling the N-isopropylamphetamine, the radioiodinated product is obtained very fast and with good radiochemical yields (Fig. 3). It can be seen that within five minutes the product is obtained with a radiochemical yield of 95%. The labelling procedure in detail is as follows: The solution containing ^{123}I-iodide in 0.01 N NaOH ist evaporated to dryness, 100 µl glacial acetic acid with 200 µg p-iodo-N-isopropylamphetamine and 2 µl of a 0.1% CuCl-solution are added and heated at 170 °C for

20 minutes. Purification of the product is performed by radio highpressure liquid chromatography using a 25 cm long stainless steel column (0.4 cm inner diameter) filled with Lichrosorb Si 60, 10 μm (Merck, Darmstadt, FRG). With a mixture of heptane/diethylamine (100/0.3) the product is eluted with a k' value of 2. Afterwards the eluens is evaporated, the product dissolved in physiological phosphate buffer (pH 7.4) and the solution is sterilized by filtration with a 0.22 μm pore size filter.

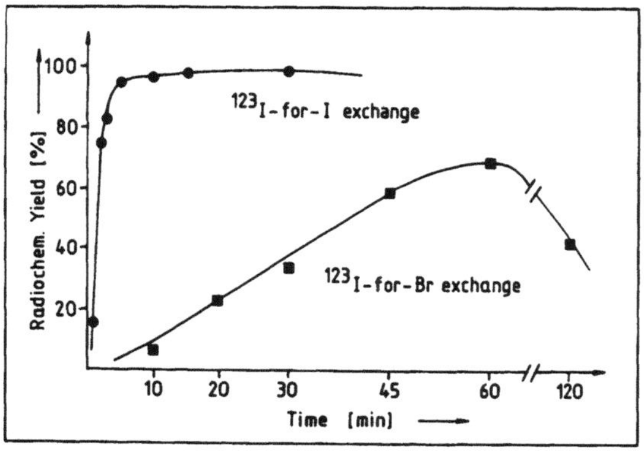

Fig. 3 Time dependence of radiochemical yields of p-^{123}I-N-isopropylamphetamine for isotope and Br exchange.

Since the ^{123}I is used in its anionic form and no oxidizing agent is present for transforming the iodine into the cationic form necessary for an electrophilic reaction mechanism, it can be assumed that the isotope exchange proceeds via a nucleophilic type of reaction. The hypothesis is supported by the applied high temperature, which is known to force the reaction from the easily proceeding electrophilic substitution to a nucleophilic reaction mechanism. If this is true, a bromine substitution by radioiodide should be possible, too, under the same reaction conditions. In p-bromo-N-isopropylamphetamine the radioiodination can indeed be performed with good radiochemical yields, as shown in Fig. 3. The product is obtained with a yield of 70% within a reaction time of one hour. Due to the higher bond energy of the bromine and the possibly higher activation energy for the substitution the reaction is slower than that of the isotope exchange. The Br-substitution by radioiodide opens the possibility to prepare IMP in very high specific activities, since by means of highpressure liquid chromatography the product can be separated from the brominated starting compound.

By the described procedures amphetamine and different N-alkylated derivatives could also be labelled with ^{123}I with similar radiochemical yields [11].

Conclusion

Within the past decade two important groups of radiopharmaceuticals labelled with ^{123}I were introduced into the clinical application opening new areas of metabolic studies in nuclear medicine:

1. by Machulla et al. [12, 13] radioiodinated fatty acids were developed for metabolic studies of the myocardium and
2. by Baldwin and coworkers [5, 6] radioiodinated amphetamine derivatives were prepared for studying brain diseases by means of SPECT

It must be emphasized that the radiochemical problems with both groups of compounds are practically the same since both are radioiodinated by a nucleophilic substitution mechanism using ^{123}I directly in its anionic form.

The clinical application of brain imaging agents, particularly the one of p-^{123}I-iodo-N-isopropylamphetamine, is important and will presumably increase as soon as the details of the individual biochemical steps, which are involved in brain uptake mechanisms, are evaluated. It is felt that the potential of the clinical IMP application is greater than the recent use of this radiopharmaceutical.

Acknowledgements

The authors would like to thank Prof. J. Rassow and Prof. C. Streffer for their generous support and interest throughout this work. Thanks are also due to Mrs. Chr. Astfalk and Mr. K. Dutschka for their valuable experimental assistance throughout this work and the team of our Compact Cyclotron for performing the irradiations.

References

[1] Machulla, H.-J., E. J. Knust: Recent developments in the field of ^{123}I-radiopharmaceuticals. Nucl.-Med. **23** (1984) 111-118.

[2] R. Weinreich: Critical comparison of production methods for ^{123}I. In: ^{123}I in Western Europe. Proceedings of a panel discussion (S. M. Quaim, G. Stöcklin, R. Weinreich, Eds.), Jül.-Conf.-20: 49–69, 1976.

[3] Reichmann, K., H. J. Biersack, G. Friedrich et al.: Significance of high energy radiation of ^{124}I or ^{123}I for brain SPECT with iodo-amphetamines. Nuc. Comp. **15** (1984) 302–304.

[4] Quaim, S. M., G. Stöcklin, R. Weinreich, Eds.: ^{123}I in Western Europe. Proceedings of a panel discussion held at KFA Jülich on February 13, 1976. Jül.-Conf.-20, 1976.

[5] Winchell, H. S., R. M. Baldwin, T. H. Lin: Development of ^{123}I labeled amines for brain studies: Localisation of ^{123}I-iodophenylalkyl amines in rat brain. J. Nucl. Med. **21** (1980) 940–946.

[6] Winchell, H. S., W. D. Horst, L. Braun et al.: N-isopropyl-[^{123}I]p-iodoamphetamine: Single-pass brain uptake and washout: Binding to brain synaptosomes and localization in dog and monkey brain. J. Nucl. Med. **21** (1980) 947–952.

[7] Kuhl, D. E., J. R. Barrio, S.-C. Huang et al.: Quantifying local cerebral blood flow by N-isopropyl-p-[^{123}I]-iodoamphetamine (IMP) tomography. J. Nucl. Med. **23** (1982) 196–203.

[8] R. M. Baldwin. This book.

[9] Machulla, H.-J.: Radioactive labelling of fatty acids for metabolic studies. In: Applications of nuclear and radiochemistry. (R. M. Lambrecht, N. Morcos, Eds.) Pergamon Press, New York. pp. 325–341, 1982.

[10] M. Eisenhut: Simple labeling of ω-phenylfatty acids by iodine isotope exchange. Int. J. Appl. Radiat. Isot. **33** (1982) 499–504.

[11] Machulla, H.-J., E. J. Knust: J. Radioanal. Nucl. Chem. (in press).

[12] Machulla, H.-J., G. Stöcklin, Ch. Kupfernagel et al.: Comparative evaluation of fatty acids labelled with ^{11}C, ^{34m}Cl. ^{77}Br and ^{123}I for metabolic studies of the myocardium: Concise communication. J. Nucl. Med. **19** (1978) 298–302.

[13] Machulla, H.-J., M. Marsmann, K. Dutschka: Biochemical concept and synthesis of a radioiodinated phenylfatty acid for in vivo metabolic studies of the myocardium. Eur. J. Nucl. Med. **5** (1980) 171–173.

Receptors for Amphetamines

R. M. Baldwin, Tz-Hong Lin, Jiann-Long Wu, J. F. Lamb

It is well known that N-isopropyl-p-iodoamphetamine (IMP) is rapidly extracted from the blood and is retained in the brain for extended periods of time [1]. Of a series of about 40 iodinated phenylalkyl amines we originally tested in the period 1977–1978 [2], IMP and its closely related structures had the highest brain uptake and retention (fig. 1). At the time, we postulated the presence of "non-specific, high-

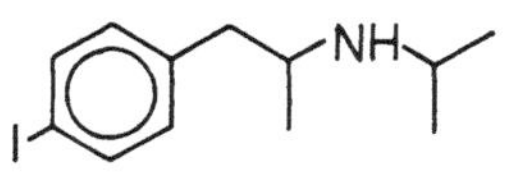

N-Isopropyl-p-iodoamphetamine

Iofetamine

IMP

Fig. 1 IMP.

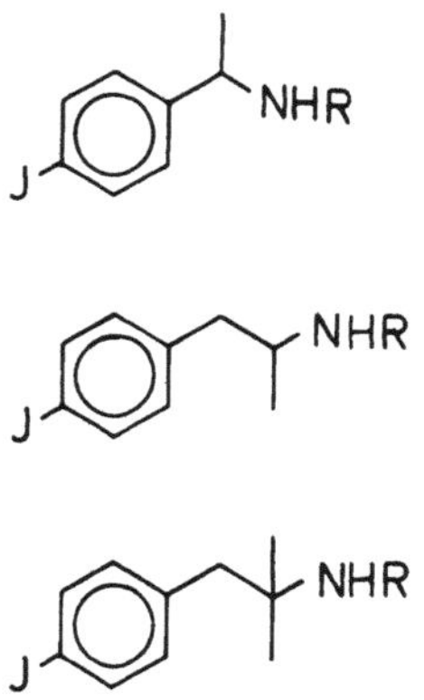

Fig. 2 Structures retained in the brain.

capacity binding sites" as a mechanism for the retention of these amines in rat brain. Our reasoning was based on the following data. First, initial brain *uptake* was similar for all the amines studied and was not dependent on the lipophilicity or basicity of the amine. Second, the *retention* of activity in brain was a function of the structure of the amine. One structural requirement for brain retention was the presence of a substituent on the carbon alpha to the nitrogen atom of the amine (fig. 2). Thus, alpha-methylbenzylamine derivatives as well as amphetamine and phentermine derivatives displayed retention [3], whereas the corresponding straight chain compounds washed out from the brain. The other important structural feature was para substitution of the aromatic ring (tab. 1). Those compounds with a para substituent showed either no decrease or a slight increase in brain activity between 5 minutes and 1 hour, whereas those compounds with an unsubstituted para position demonstrated a drop in the activity in brain with time. A third considera-tion which argued for a binding mechanism was the observation that IMP displaced serotonin from brain synaptosomes [4].

Table 1 Effect of substitution pattern on brain retention

Position	% Isomeric Purity	% Dose/g Brain 5 min	60 min	Brain/Blood Ratio 5 min	60 min
ortho	92	1.0	0.6	8.2	7.0
meta	44	1.1	0.9	3.1	6.5
para	98	1.5	1.9	10.3	12.2
di-iodo	99	1.1	1.2	8.7	11.0

These results suggested that a simple physicochemical explanation such as lipophilicity was not sufficient to explain the brain retention of these amines. Yet, specific receptor binding could not be the explanation, either. First, the brain uptake was non-saturatable: within experimental limits, there was no change in brain uptake between carrier doses of carrier-free up to 0.5 mg per kg. Second, uptake was not specific for optical configuration (tab. 2). The uptake and retention of the different optical isomers of either IMP or its dealkylated counterpart p-iodoamphetamine were similar. Specific receptors would be expected to behave steroselectively.

Table 2 Effect of optical configuration on brain retention

Compound	Configuration	% Dose/g Brain 5 min	60 min	Brain/Blood Ratio 5 min	60 min
PIA	R (−)	1.4	2.1	10.6	18.5
	S (+)	1.2	1.9	7.0	11.3
IMP	R (−)	1.7	1.9	15.8	20.0
	S (+)	1.5	2.1	11.4	16.1
	RS (±)	1.5	1.9	10.3	12.2

Dr. Blau and Kung, in some elegant reasoning, have rationalized the action of another series of radiolabeled amines in terms of what has been called the "pH shift hypothesis" [5]. Briefly, this suggests that the preferential retention of labeled amines is due to the pH gradient that exists between the plasma (pH 7.4) and the brain (pH 7.0). Thus, the concentration of unionized (lipophilic) amine will be greater in the plasma than in the brain, allowing free diffusion into the brain, whereas in the more acidic medium of the brain, the material will exist more in the ionized (lipophobic) form, and will be impeded from diffusing out of the brain. Implicit in this treatment is that the unionized free base is lipophilic, whereas the ionized form is not. The differential retention of amines would then be explained by the narrow requirements for having a basicity in the right range to benefit from the "pH shift" effect. Indeed, in radio-selenium labeled amines, the observed behavior correlated well with that predicted from theory [6].

We explored the possibility of "pH shift" as a possible mechanism for the brain uptake and retention of amphetamines and related compounds [7]. We measured the octanol-buffer partition coefficients (PC) of representative members of our series as a function of pH and compared the PC/pH profile to the brain uptake and retention observed in rats. If "pH shift" were dominant, then we would expect those compounds with high brain retention to exhibit different PC/pH profiles from those compounds that were not retained. Such was not the case, however. Although the compounds did display a range of behavior (fig. 3), there was no relation between the PC/pH profile and the brain uptake and retention. For instance, N-t-butyl-o-iodobenzylamine had a profile almost identical to that of IMP; however, the benzylamine derivative washed out from the brain within one hour, whereas IMP activity increased over the same time period. On the other extreme, p-iodoamphetamine, which displayed similar brain retention to that of IMP, had a distinctly different profile; yet, the ortho isomer o-iodoamphetamine, with a similar profile to p-iodoamphetamine, washed out from the brain. Furthermore, the partition coefficients of these amines even at acidic pH were well above the threshold value of about 0.5 for essentially complete extraction by the brain [8]. We therefore concluded that, at least in the series of amines we have tested, the "pH shift" hypothesis cannot explain their long term retention.

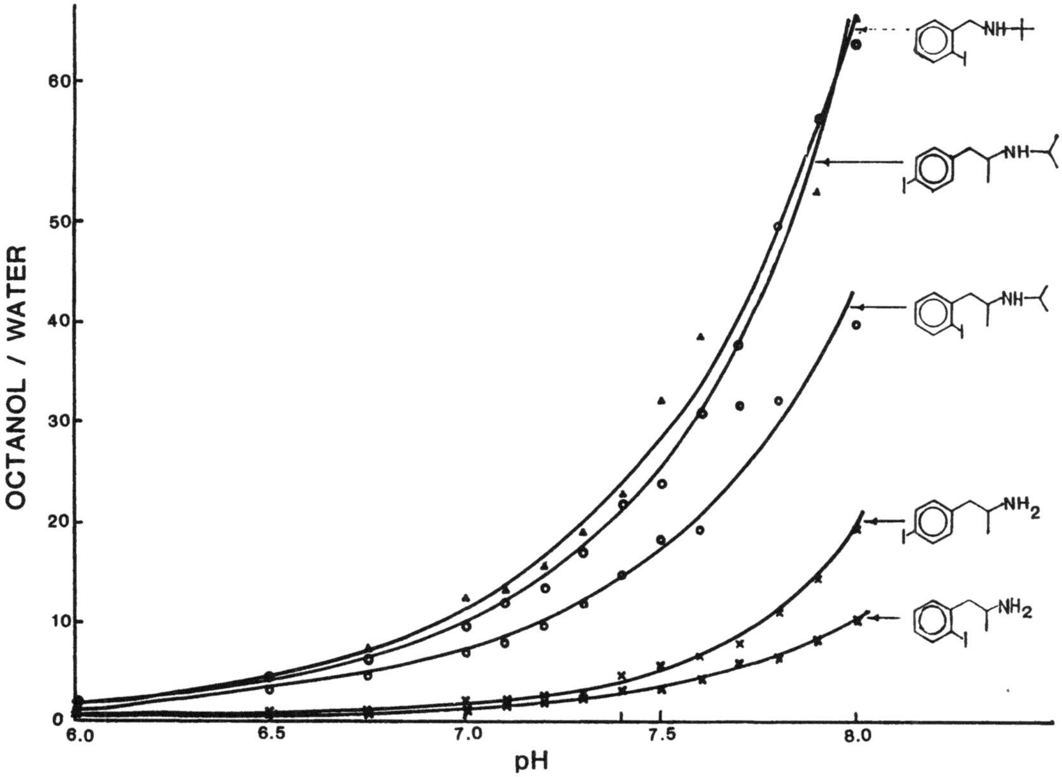

Fig. 3 PC-pH profiles of iodinated amines.

We return to the concept of "high-capacity non-specific" binding. This is largely a hand-waving argument, descriptive of the phenomenon without explaining it: a relatively large amount of IMP can be taken up and retained by the brain, hence the system has a "high capacity", and there appears to be a wide latitude of structural variation, hence "non-specific". Is the concept of such a binding mechanism reasonable? The following evidence suggests the possibility of a binding system for amines in the *lungs* which fulfills the requirement for high capacity. This work was conducted by Dr. J. J. Touya at the VA Hospital in Fresno and Dr. L. R. Bennett at the University of California at Los Angeles, California.

The experiments were carried out in African pygmy goats, which have a chest anatomy approximating that found in man. ^{123}I labeled IMP was injected intravenously with reference tracers to correct for vascular and extravascular activity in the region of the lungs; activity was measured with a gamma counter and the computer was used to calculate count rates as a function of time [9]. Measured quantities of carrier IMP were then coinjected in a series of experiments and the effect on the lung extraction of labeled IMP was measured. On addition of carrier IMP, lung extraction was reduced by a factor of up to 5. A classical Scatchard plot demonstrated the saturability of this system, and the affinity could be calculated as 30 mg IMP in the lung of the animal at half saturation [10]. This represents a high capacity system. Furthermore, other amines, such as ketamine, propanolol, and guanethidine, displaced IMP, demonstrating non-specificity. In the lungs, at least, then, the concept of non-specific, high-capacity binding mechanisms has been shown to be a reasonable hypothesis.

It may be that the reason saturation has not been observed in the brain is that the capacity is greater than the largest amount of material that can be practically administered to the animals. We are also exploring the possibility that differential metabolism of amines in the brain could explain the results, since para substitution would block para hydroxylation, a major route of amphetamine metabolism [11], and alpha methylation would be expected to hinder oxidative attack at the amino function [12].

References

[1] Holman, B. L., T. C. Hill, R. G. L. Lee et al.: Brain imaging with radiolabeled amines. In: Nuclear Medicine Annual 1983 (Freeman, L. M., Weissman, H. S., Eds.). Raven Press, pp. 131–165, 1983.

[2] Winchell, H. S., R. M. Baldwin, T. H. Lin: Development of ^{123}I labeled amines for brain studies: Localization of ^{123}I-iodophenylalkyl amines in rat brain. J. Nucl. Med. **21** (1980) 940–946.

[3] Lin, T. H., R. M. Baldwin, J. L. Wu et al.: Development of ^{123}I-N-isopropyl-p-iodoamphetamine: Exploration, synthesis, and metabolism. 16th Japan Conf. Rad. Radioisot. Tokyo, December 6.–8., 1983.

[4] Winchell, H. S., W. D. Horst, L. Braun. et al.: N-Isopropyl-[^{123}I]-p-iodoamphetamine: Single-pass brain uptake and washout; binding to brain synaptosomes; and localization in dog and monkey brain. J. Nucl. Med. **21** (1980) 947–952.

[5] Tramposch, K. M., H. F. Kung, M. Blau.: Brain imaging with ^{123}I labeled diamines: a kit preparation suitable for routine clinical use. J. Nucl. Med. **22** (1981) 12.
[6] Kung, H. F., M. Blau.: Regional intracellular pH shift: a proposed new mechanism for radiopharmaceutical uptake in brain and other tissues. J. Nuc. Med. **21** (1980) 147–152.
[7] Lin, T. H., B. M. Mar, J. L. Wu et al.: Brain Localization and octanol/water PC-pH profiles of radioiodinated amines: Evidence against "pH shift". J. Nucl. Med. **25** (1984) 122.
[8] Oldendorf, W. H.: Lipid solubility and drug penetration of the blood brain barrier (38444). Proc. Soc. Exp. Biol. Med. **147** (1974) 813–816.
[9] Rahimian, J., L. R. Bennett, D. Grubbs et al.: A noninvasive procedure to measure in vivo lung endothelial receptors. J. Nucl. Med. **24** (1983) 71.
[10] Rahimian, J. R., E. C. Glass, J. J. Touya et al.: Measurement of metabolic extraction of tracers in the lung using a multiple indicator dilution technique. J. Nucl. Med. **25** (1984) 31–37.
[11] Lemberger, L., A. Rubin: Amphetamine. In: Physiologic Disposition of Drugs of Abuse. Spectrum Publishers, N. Y., pp. 31–63, 1976.
[12] Caldwell, J.: The metabolism of amphetamines and related stimulants in animals and man. In: Amphetamines and Related Stimulants: Chemical, Biological, Clinical, and Sociological Aspects. CRC Press, Boca Raton, FL, pp. 29–46, 1980.

Metabolism of Amphetamines

G. Pfeiffer

The metabolism of radioiodinated alkylated amphetamines like N-isopropyl-p-iodo-amphetamine (IMP) is based on the pharmacokinetics and on the metabolism of amphetamines, which have been intensively studied since years. A first summary was given by Vree in 1973 [1]. In this paper a short review will demonstrate the very controversary data published till now.

Biodistribution and unaltered excretion

After ingestion or intravenous administration of amphetamines or one of its derivatives the compound will be distributed in the body. The distribution volume of amphetamine-hydrochloride lies between 200–300 ml, N-alkylated amphetamines show smaller volumes of about 50 ml and therefore a higher blood level. The excretion rate in the urine is linearily dependent on the blood concentration: after ingestion of 1 mg amphetamine (a dose, used in nuclear medicine) the blood level is in the range of 3-7 µg/ml and the excretion rate in the urine about 1 µg/ml. If amphetamines are in a neutral, non polar form, they can be reabsorbed. At pH 7.4 (the physiologic variation of urinary pH is 4.7–7.5) only 0.3% are in this neutral form, at pH 5 only 0.003%. Therefore the main amount of amphetamine will be excreted unaltered. Concerning IMP, the N-alkyl group shifts the molecule in the non polar direction, but this effect will be compensated by the halogen atom, which shifts in the opposite direction (N-isopropyl-amphetamine 0.18% neural at pH 7, p-chloro-amphetamine 0.39%), so that in summary IMP shows excretion rates similar to amphetamine [1].

Metabolism

Besides this first pathway of metabolism, the unaltered excretion, amphetamines will be transformed to more polar compounds by different mechanisms. In fig. 1 the starting points of 4 different pathways are marked at the general formula of amphetamines. The intermediates and the resulting endproducts of these reactions are subsequently described.

(1) 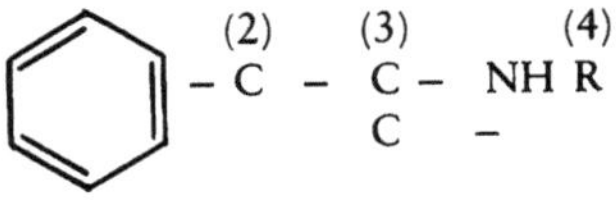

(1) parahydroxylation
(2) β–C–hydroxylation
(3) α–C–desamination
(4) N-dealkylation

Fig. 1 Amphetamines: starting points for metabolism.

Para-hydroxylation

This reaction is very common in the metabolism of various lipophilic drugs. Axelrod [2] injected 5 mg/kg amphetamine to various animal species and found in the urine of rats and dogs para-hydroxy-amphetamine (p-OH-AMP) to a significant amount, while in the rabbit and in the guinea pig neither hydroxylated nor unaltered AMP was excreted. The p-OH-AMP is excreted partly free or conjugated with sulfuric or glucuronic acid. If p-OH-AMP was administered to these animals, it was excreted to more than 40% in all of them. In table 1 Axelrods data are summarized.

Table 1 Excretion of D-amphetamine and D-p-OH-amphetamine [2]

Species	Ingestion of D-AMP Excretion of		Ingestion of D-p-OH-AMP Excretion of
	D-AMP (%)	p-OH-AMP (%)	p-OH-AMP (%)
Dog	31.0	20.0	61
Rat	13.0	31.0	38
Guinea pig	0.7	0.5	69
Rabbit	1.2	3.6	55

Beta-hydroxylation

This metabolic process is catalyzed by the steric specific enzyme betahydroxylase and takes place in the brain. This pathway is less important for catabolism than for pharmacological effects, because the resulting compounds belong to the group of ephedrines and can easily undergo further transformations to epinephrines or, in special cases, to catecholamines. Fig. 2 demonstates the close chemical relation between these four groups of biologic active amines.

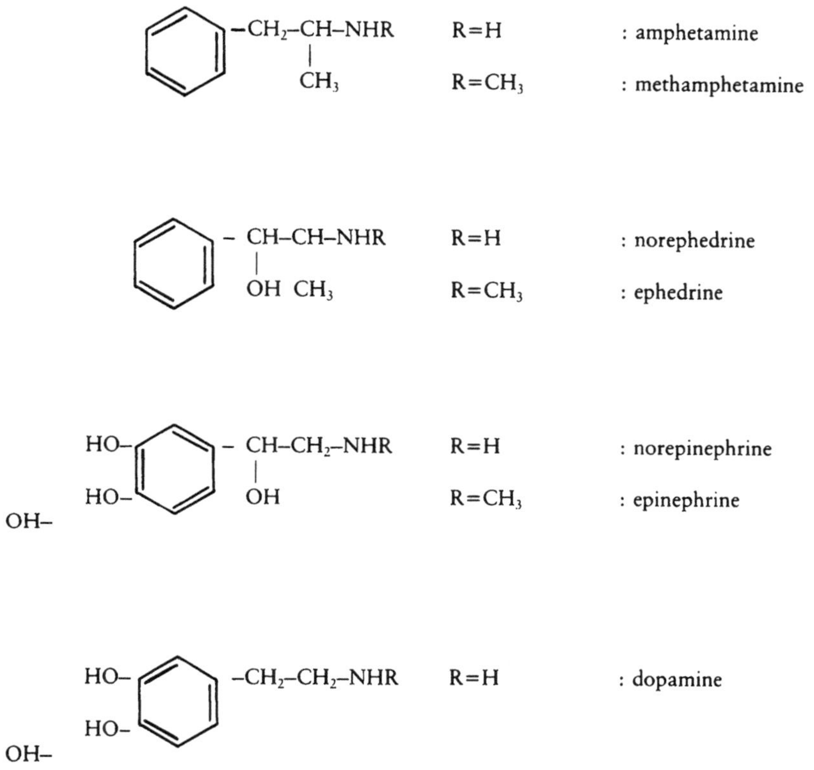

Fig. 2 Amphetamines–ephedrines–epinephrines–catecholamines.

The conversion to ephedrines may be responsible for the occurence of strange effects, observed after administration of radiolabelled alkylated amphetamines like the second rise of blood activity.

In the rat p-OH-AMP is accumulated by cortical and striatal synaptosomes. The brain microsomes contain a cytochrome-P-450 dependent monooxygenase (MAO) which synthesizes catecholamines from p-OH-AMP. The formation of this metabolite may be involved in the development of tolerance in chronic amphetamine use [3].

Desamination

This reaction is the main pathway in man and starts with the addition of a hydroxylgroup to the α-carbon atom. This intermediate is desaminated and oxidized to the ketone either on a direct or an indirect way, as fig. 3 shows.

The desamination always includes bioinactivation. The resulting ketone, phenylpropanone, will be further metabolized to benzoic acid which is excreted in the urine as benzoic acid or, coupled with glycin, as hippuric acid.

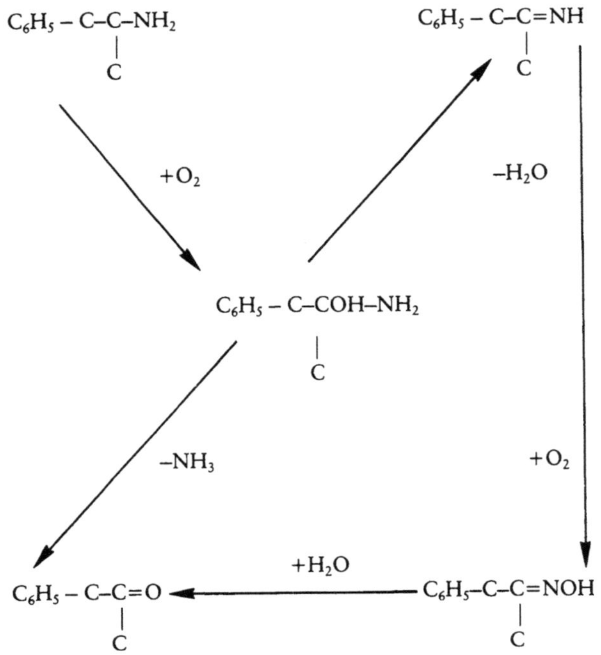

Fig. 3 Desamination.

Dring [4] determined the metabolites of carbon-14-labelled amphetamine in different species. The determination of the metabolites in the urine was performed by isotope dilution analysis. His data, summarized in tab. 2 show the percentual portion of the three pathways (unaltered excretion, para-hydroxylation and desamination) on the total excretion. Only in the rabbit the ketone was found in the urine. Compared to Axelrods data the individual values are not in total agreement (Drings analytical technique is more sensitive), but the statements are similar: in the dog the main excretion way is the unaltered excretion, in the rat the parahydroxylation and in the rabbit the desamination.

In a ^{14}C-balance study on humans Dring found a very good agreement between the sum of identified metabolites and the total ^{14}C-excretion. He looked at the influence

Table 2 Metabolites of ^{14}C-AMP in different species [4]

Species Dose (mg/kg)	man 0.07	rhesus 0.66	dog 5	rabbit 10	rat 10	mouse 10	guin. 5
amphetamine	30	31	30	4	13	33	22%
p-OH-amphetamine	3	11	6	6	60	14	0
benzoic acid	21	31	28	25	3	31	62
phenylpropanone	3	0	2	29	0	0	0
total	57	73	66	64	76	78	84

of the steric configuration on the excretion mode, too. As tab. 3 shows, the excretion rate during 24 h is about 60% for all three isomers (65, 58, 66%) and the main excreted compound is unaltered amphetamine. Little differences in the excretion mode between the three isomers could be observed in humans and in animals, too.

Table 3 Metabolites of ^{14}C-AMP in human urine [4]

Metabolites	(+)-AMP	(−)-AMP	(±)-AMP
amphetamine	34.0	34.0	30.0%
p-OH-AMP	1.1	3.9	2.8
benzoic acid	21.0	13.0	21.0
phenylacetone	2.2	1.3	3.4
sum	58.0	52.0	57.0
^{14}C total (24 h)	65.0	58.0	66.0

More impressive than the differences due to the steric configuration are the individual differences: in the urine of one person considerable amounts of p-OH-AMP could be detected, which was totally absent in the other two. A similar effect could be observed in rhesus monkeys.

The role of enzymes involved in this process was investigated by various scientists. Parly [5] found, that the direct and the indirect reaction to the ketone in rat liver microsomes are cytochrome-P-450 dependent and catalized by microsomal monooxygenases and TPNH as cofactor. Blume [6] used highly purified liver mitochondria. He prooved the essential role of NADPH but failed to detect cytochrome-P-450. In vitro studies by Matsumoto [7] indicate that N-hydroxy-AMP is transformed by rat liver homogenates to phenylacetone-oxime. This oxidation is NADPH and oxygen dependent, but cytochrome P-450 was not necessary for this reaction. The oxime is the precursor of phenylacetone. In comparison to Parlys work there is more than one pathway from AMP to the resulting ketone, depending on the species (rabbit/rat). The high affinity of some drugs (Haloperidol, Diazepam) to these enzymes explains their inhibitory effect on amphetamines.

Dealkylation

The dealkylation process of alkylated amphetamines is performed in the liver using oxydizing enzymes. Desamination and desalkylation are competitive reactions. The selection of the main way is given by the character of the substituent (straight or branched chain) and the steric configuration. Comparing to pure AMP all alkylated amphetamines show longer half lives in the blood (p. e. AMP 7 h, Captagon 10 h). The L-forms are usually less sensitive to the desamination process due to the steric specificity of the enzymes. Three different mechanisms are considered [1]: in one process a nitrogen-oxide works as in intermediate, the other two are oxydative mechanisms (proton split off or addition of oxygen), analogue to the desamination process.

The simplest alkylated amphetamine, N-methyl-AMP, was investigated by Axelrod [2]. In the dog he found an unaltered excretion of 18% and a demethylation rate of about 45%. The resulting AMP was excreted partly unaltered and partly in the form of 4-OH-AMP as described before. Coutts [8] investigated the in vivo metabolism of N-alkylated amphetamines in the rat. According to Axelrod he found, following the administration of amphetamine and methylamphetamine, only one phenolic metabolite, namely p-OH-AMP, but, as the length of the N-alkylchain increases, a second metabolite, 4-hydroxy-3-methoxyAMP in a significant amount. This metabolite again demonstrates the close relation of amphetamines and catecholamines.

Systematic studies on various mono- and di-alkylated amphetamines in humans were undertaken by Donike [9]. After dosing with 10 mg the cumulative excretion was determined during 24 h and the separation between original compound and metabolites was done by gaschromatography. The non-substituted AMP was excreted to about 60%. Concerning the derivatives the authors found a linear relation between cumulative excretion, number of carbon atoms and lipid solubility. Dialkylated amphetamines are desalkylated in two steps: very quickly desalkylation to the mono-alkylated compound and the second step, corresponding to the kinetics of the monoalkylated amine. An analogous study was published by Testa [10]: he tested 15 alkylated amphetamines and found a very fast excretion of tertiary amines, followed by the secondary and, at least, the primary amines.

The qualitative and quantitative aspects of the urinary elimination of 4-methoxy-AMP (^{14}C-labelled) has been examined in rats, guinea pigs and humans by Kitchen [11]. In all three species O-demethylation to 4-OH-AMP was the main metabolic pathway. Side chain oxydation to 1(4'methoxy phenyl)propane-2-one oxime occured in the guinea pig and to a small amount in humans, too. Marked intersubject variations could be observed. In dogs and monkeys Midha [12] found 3-Methoxy-α-methyldopamine in the urine after ingestion of mescaline or TMA (methoxy derivatives of AMP). These derivatives show a direct relation to the catecholamines.

Elimination

In the metabolism of secondary amphetamines the elimination is due to excretion of the unaltered compound, the desamination and the N-dealkylation. The parahydroxylation may be neglected in humans. In tab. 4 the percentual portions of these three pathways are listed for three pairs (optical isomers) of amphetamines [1], which show significant differences.

D-N-isopropylamphetamine is rapidly eliminated from the body with a half life of 2–3 h, because the metabolite D-AMP is formed very fast. The L-isomer on the contrary is excreted mainly unaltered (90%) and is hardely metabolized.

Table 4 Elimination = excretion + desamination + dealkylation [1]

	excretion (%)	desamination (%)	dealkylation (%)
(+) amphetamine	70	30	–
(−) amphetamine	90	10	–
(+) N-methyl-AMP	65	20	15
(−) N-methyl-AMP	80	10	10
(+) N-isopropyl-AMP	10	45	45
(−) N-isopropyl-AMP	85	0	15

Differences between the optical isomers were observed by Ames, too [13], who studied the metabolism of p-chloro-amphetamine in rabbit liver microsomal preparations. NADPH and molecular oxygen are necessary for this process, which was more rapidly in the R than in the S isomer, and more rapidly, if these isomers are incubated individually than if incubated as part of the racemic mixture.

Iodine-labelled amphetamines (IMP)

During the development of N-isopropyl-p-iodoamphetamine, labelled with ^{123}I, Winchell [14] studied more than 20 different iodinated amphetamine derivatives in respect of brain uptake and blood to brain ratio. His tests showed that the optimal substituent was isopropyl and the iodine had to be in para position. The progressive increase of radioactivity in the stomach of rats Winchell explained by the in vivo deiodination and the accumulation of radioiodide in the gastric mucosa, according to the pH gradient. The body distribution and the metabolites of IMP in the urine of the rat were investigated by Rapin [15]. He found besides the wellknown activity concentration in lungs, liver and brain significant amounts of radioiodine in the gastrointestinal tract and a thyroid uptake of 0.03%. The urine was analyzed for amines, desaminated and hydroxylated compounds and acid derivatives. His results (tab. 5) show a time shift of metabolism: in the beginning unaltered excretion, lateron desamination to benzoic acid.

In monkeys Holman [16] determined the thyroid uptake in unblocked thyroids of maximal 0.25%. This value remained constant from day 1 to day 5. He, too,

Table 5 Metabolites from IMP in rat urine [15]

	0–6 h	6–24 h	24–48 h
amines	61 ± 5	23 ± 4	14 ± 2
desaminated	29 ± 3	39 ± 2	30 ± 1
acids	10 ± 3	38 ± 3	56 ± 10

assumes a break down of IMP and discusses the N-dealkylation and the beta-hydroxylation as possible metabolic pathways.

In men, the unblocked thyroid was faintly seen. Delaloye [17] estimated an uptake of about 1% from his total body scans. Kuhl [18] investigated the distribution of IMP in human blood. His studies showed that IMP was freely exchangeable between red cells and plasma. No metabolism of IMP occured within the red cells, only IMP was found by HPLC. In the arterial blood some unidentified polar metabolites could be detected. In the human urine Kuhl identified by thin layer chromatography unmodified IMP, p-iodo-amphetamine, p-iodo-phenylacetone, p-iodo-benzoic acid, p-iodo-hippuric acid and free iodide. This analysis gives evidence, that N-desalkylation is the first and desamination the second metabolic step in IMP metabolism in humans.

Moretti [19] tried to get some data about the parmacokinetics of IMP. He found an increase of the plasma activity in relation to total blood activity with time. About one hour after injection the first polar metabolites appear in the plasma and 24 h post injection the total plasma activity consists of polar metabolites (tab. 6). Moretti only separated polar from nonpolar compounds by resin without identification of the various substances.

Table 6 IMP-metabolism in blood [19]

	3 h	6 h	24 h	48 h
blood cells (% dose)	0.28	0.27	0.25	0.29
plasma (% dose)	0.77	1.39	1.80	1.65
IMP in plasma (%)	0.60	1.01	0.88	0.80
metabolites plasma (%)	0.17	0.38	0.92	0.85

Other labelled amphetamines, like HIPDM are metabolized in a similar way: after N-dealkylation by an N-methyltransferase the desamination follows, catalyzed by monoaminooxidase or diaminooxidase [20].

In the lung, where various sorts of biogenic amines are trapped, IMP will be trapped, too, and partly removed by oxidative deamination, catalyzed by MAO enzymes.

Summary

Some important points of the metabolism of amphetamines will be summarized and their consequences for the metabolism of the radiopharmaceutical N-isopropyl-p-iodo (^{123}I)-amphetamine (IMP) according to Winchells paper lined out [14]:

(1) Dependent on the pH of the urine significant amounts of unaltered substance will be excreted.

(2) The competition between desamination and dealkylation will be influenced by the length and form of the side chain and the steric configuration. The endproducts of the desamination are benzoic and hippuric acid or the iodinated derivatives.

(3) The betahydroxylation in the brain transforms the amphetamines to derivatives of ephedrines or epinephrines, which show high biologic activity and may be responsible for brain retention.

(4) The para-hydroxylation, not a main pathway in humans, will be blocked by the iodine in para position in the case of IMP.

(5) The methylgroup on the α-carbon will inhibit the activity of oxidative enzymes.

References

[1] Vree, T. B.: Pharmacokinetics and metabolism of amphetamines. Thesis, Univ. of Nijmegen, Dept. Pharmacology, 1973.

[2] Axelrod, J.: Studies on sympathomimetic amines. II the biotransformation and physiological disposition of D-amphetamine, D-p-hydroxyamphetamine and D-methamphetamine. J. Pharm. Exp. Ther. **110** (1954) 315.

[3] Hoffman, A. R., B. V. Sastry, J. Axelrod: Formation of alpha-methyldopamine ("catecholamphetamine") from p-hydroxy-amphetamine by rat brain microsomes. Pharmacology **19** (1979) 256.

[4] Dring, L. G., R. L. Schmidt, R. T. Williams: The metabolic fate of amphetamine in man and other species. Biochem. J. **116** (1970) 425.

[5] Parly, C. J., N. Wang, R. E. McMahon: The enzymatic N-hydroxylation of an imine. J. biol. chem. **246** (1971) 6953.

[6] Blume, H.: Biotransformation von Amphetaminderivaten durch Rattenlebermitochondrien, I Oxidative Entalkylierung von N,N-dialkyl- und N-alkylamphetaminen und II Oxidative Desaminierung von Amphetamin und Reduktion von Phenylaceton. Arzneimittelforschung (Drug. Res.) **31** (1981) 805 and 994.

[7] Matsumoto, R. M., A. K. Cho: Conversion of N-hydroxyamphetamine to phenylacetone oxime by rat liver microsomes. Biochem. Pharmacol. **31** (1982) 105.

[8] Coutts, R. T., G. W. Dawson, G. R. Jones: In vivo metabolism of N-alkyl-ampetamines in the rat – the effect of N-alkyl chain length on oxidation of the aromatic ring. Res. Commun. Chem. Pathol. Pharmacol. **22** (1978) 589.

[9] Donike, M., R. Iffland, L. Jaenicke: Der Einfluß der N-Alkylgruppe auf die N-Dealkylierungsgeschwindigkeit bei N-Alkyl- und N,N-Dialkylamphetaminderivaten in vivo. Arzneim. Forsch. (Drug. Res.) **24** (1974) 556.

[10] Testa, B., B. Salvesen: Quantitative structure-activity relationship in drug metabolism and disposition: Pharmacokinetics of N-substituted amphetamines in humans. J. Pharm. Sci. **69** (1980) 497.

[11] Kitchen, I., J. Tremblay, J. Andre et al.: Interindividual and interspecies variation in the metabolism of the hallucinogen 4-methoxyamphetamine. Xenobiotica **9** (1979) 397.

[12] Midha, K. K., K. Bailey, J. K. Cooper et al.: Metabolic O-demethylation of 3,4-dimethoxyamphetamine in vivo in dog and monkey. Xenobiotica **9** (1979) 485.

[13] Ames, M. M., S. K. Frank: Stereochemical aspects of para-chloramphetamine metabolism. Rabbit liver microsomal metabolism of RS,R(−) and S(i-para-chloramphetamine). Biochem. Pharmacol. **31** (1982) 5.

[14] Winchell, H. S., R. M. Baldwin, T. H. Lin: Development of ^{123}I labelled amines for brain studies: localization of ^{123}I-iodophenylalkylamines in rat brain. J. Nucl. Med. **21** (1980) 940.

[15] Rapin, J. R., D. Duterte, M. Leponcin-Lafitte et al.: Aspects chimique et pharmacologique des traceurs cellulaires cérébraux. Sem. Hop. Paris **59** (1983) 3361.

[16] Holman, B. L., R. E. Zimmerman, J. R. Shapiro et al.: Biodistribution and dosimetry of N-isopropyl-p(^{123}I)-iodoamphetamine in the primate. J. Nucl. Med. **24** (1983) 922.

[17] Bischof-Delaloye, A., J. P. Hungerbühler, F. Regli et al.: ^{123}I-iodoamphetamine: preliminary results on biokinetics and distribution of cerebral blood flow. Radioaktive Isotope in Klinik und Forschung, Internat. Symposium, Urban und Schwarzenberg, Band 16/1, 1984, S. 27.

[18] Kuhl, D. E., J. R. Barrio, S. C. Huang et al.: Quantifying local cerebral blood flow by N-isopropyl-p-(^{123}I)-iodoamphetamine (IMP) tomography. J. Nucl. Med. **23** (1982) 196.

[19] Moretti, J. L.: N-isopropyl-iodoamphetamine, an agent for brain imaging with SPECT. In: Functional radionuclide imaging of the brain. (Ed.: Ph. L. Magistretti), Serono Symposia Vol. 5, Raven Press, 1983, p. 231.

[20] Kung, H. F., K. T. Tramposch, M. Blau: A new brain perfusion imaging agent: ^{123}I-HIPDM. J. Nucl. Med. **24** (1983) 66.

New Amphetamine Derivatives

H. Klünenberg

In 1975 Sargent et al. [1] for the first time pointed out the possibility of using ^{77}Br-labelled amine derivatives for the brain-scintigraphy. Not until 5 years later the group Winchell and co-workers [2] reported again about these new kinds of radio-pharmaceuticals, which are able to cross the blood-brain-barrier.

In 1981 the first paper on the application of such a testing-compound on human beings came out [3]. One year later the first emission-computer-tomographic results of the Hill and Holman group were presented [4]. For about the last two years ^{123}I-labelled N-isopropyl-p-iodoamphetamine (IMP) has been used for the diagnosis of brain diseases [5–14]. ^{123}I-HIPDM, which was developed by the group of Blau and Kung [15] in 1982, showed similarly good results.

However, due to the fact that there is only 5 to 10% cerebral uptake, relatively high amounts of the ^{123}I-labelled tracer have to be administered, resulting in high costs. Above that, its extensive pulmonary retention leads to a high radiation burden to this organ.

These reasons prompted us to evaluate other tracers with superior properties for brain imaging.

We chose the amphetamine-containing psycho-pharmaceutical "Fenetylline" as a first compound [16] (fig. 1).

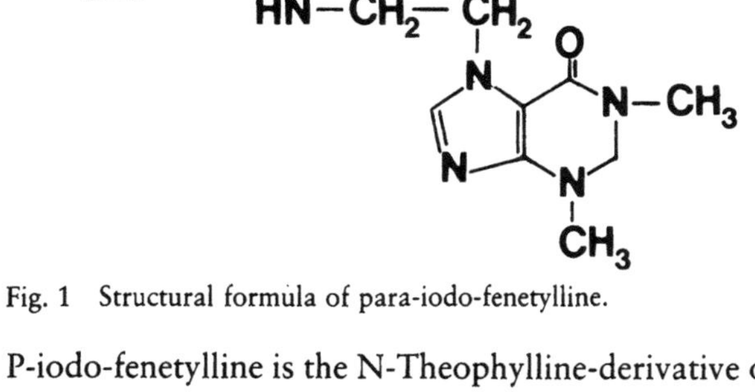

Fig. 1 Structural formula of para-iodo-fenetylline.

P-iodo-fenetylline is the N-Theophylline-derivative of p-iodoamphetamine, the non-iodinated form of which is available on the market as "Captagon".

The cold-iodinated compound was labelled in an exchange reaction with ^{131}I in an acidic, aqueous solution by means of Cu-catalysis. IMP was labelled with ^{125}I in the same way in order to have a direct comparison for the following analyses.

Table 1 Organ kinetics from 5–120 min. p. i. after simultaneous application of ^{125}I-isopropylamphetamine and ^{131}I-fenetylline in the rat

	% ^{125}I/g tissue (^{125}I-amphetamine)						% ^{131}I/g tissue (^{131}I-fenetylline)					
Organ	5′	10′	15′	30′	60′	120′	5′	10′	15′	30′	60′	120′
Brain	1.3	1.9	1.7	0.9	1.7	2.2	1.0	1.3	0.4	0.2	0.5	1.3
Cerebellum	1.7	2.1	2.0	0.7	1.4	1.9	1.2	0.7	0.4	0.1	0.4	1.2
Liver	1.4	2.5	2.9	1.5	1.7	3.4	3.8	4.0	2.0	0.8	1.1	3.4
Lung	10.6	31.8	14.1	5.3	10.5	11.7	7.9	21.3	5.0	2.3	4.8	6.8
Kidney	2.8	5.0	2.9	0.8	2.0	2.2	3.5	5.3	1.5	0.5	1.7	3.1
Spleen	1.7	1.5	2.5	1.6	1.7	2.6	2.6	2.6	1.2	0.7	0.8	2.1
Myocardium	2.2	3.9	1.0	0.4	0.7	0.7	2.3	3.8	0.8	0.3	0.7	1.0
Muscle	0.1	0.2	0.3	0.2	0.3	0.4	0.3	0.5	0.3	0.2	0.3	0.6
Urine	0.04	0.3	0.7	3.0	4.8	18.0	0.2	0.6	2.0	5.4	12.4	70.4
Blood	0.3	0.7	0.6	0.1	0.3	0.2	0.8	1.6	1.3	0.1	0.6	0.5

In a first series of tests 30 wistar-rats were injected simultaneously ^{125}I-IMP as well as ^{131}I-p-iodo-fenetylline. The animals were killed after 5, 10, 15, 30, 60 and 120 min. Afterwards the radioactivity-content in different organs was measured by a well counter.

In a second series of tests it was checked whether the simultaneous injection possibly leads to a competitive inhibition of the Fenetylline-uptake. For that purpose 10 rats were administered with ^{131}I-p-iodo-fenetylline. The proportional uptake per gram was determined after 15 and 60 min.

Tab. 1 shows the results of the organ-distribution from 5–120 min after a simultaneous dose of ^{125}I-IMP and ^{131}I-p-iodo-fenetylline.

IMP shows a quick increase in the brain tissue up to about 1.9%/gram (after 10 min), which decreases a little afterwards and then increases again up to 2.2% per gram (after 2 h). The activity in the lung shows a maximum of ~ 32% after 10 min, then passes through a minimum of 5.3% after 30 min and rises again up to 10.5% after 60 min and 11.7% after 120 min.

Biokinetics of radio-iodinated Fenetylline differs substantially from IMP: The maximum cerebral uptake is only about 1.3% per gram of tissue and decreases after 30 min and 60 min to 0.2% and 0.5% per gram of tissue respectively. The lung accumulation is not as distinct as with IMP (21.3% to 31.8%: 10 min p.i.). Also, the urine excretion of Fenetylline is substantially higher than that of IMP (70.4% to 18% per gram after 2 h). On the other hand, the blood-clearance is higher than that of Fenetylline.

From the data obtained from animals it can be concluded, that with lower cerebral incorporation of radioactivity by Fenetylline – in connection with a higher blood-radioactivity – basically the results cannot be expected to be as favourable as with the application of IMP. This assumption was proved to be correct by a sequential scintigraphy from 2 dogs.

Fig. 2 illustrates the sequential scintigraphy as well as the functional curve of a dog after i.v. application of 500 μCi ^{131}I-Fenetylline. At first the sequential scintigraphy shows a rapid uptake of radioactivity in the brain, after 10 to 15 min, however, a quick activity-decrease is to be seen.

Because of these results, which were verified by ^{123}I-Fenetylline-SPECT on three patients, further research work with this compound has been postponed for the time being. Of course, one cannot exclude the possibility of using p-iodo-fenetylline as perfusionsmarker, provided that suitable camera technique, i.e. very fast rotating equipment, is available.

During our search for a suitable substance, which will be able to cross the blood-brain-barrier, we tested 4N-alkyl-derivatives of p-iodoamphetamine, the chemical structure of which can be seen in fig. 3.

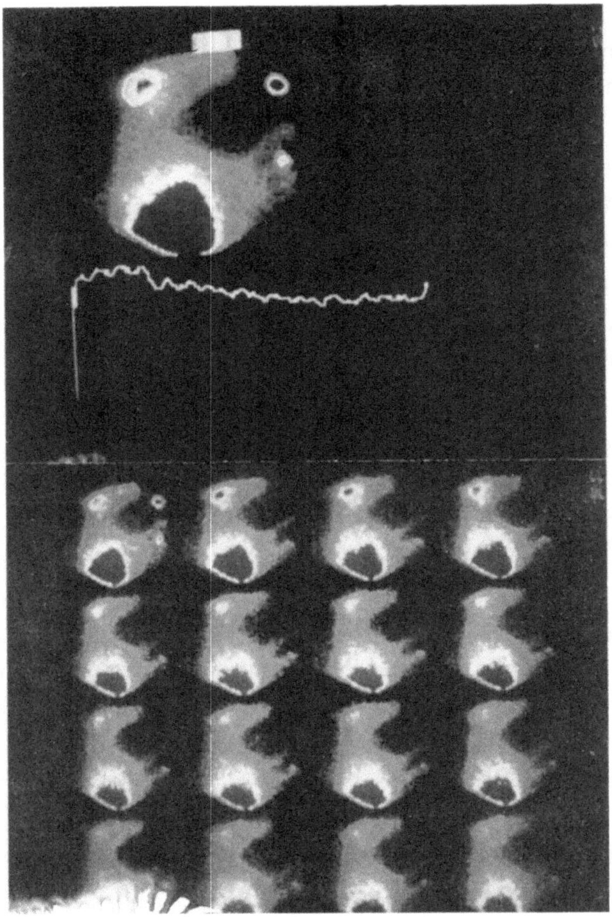

Fig. 2 Histogram (upper) and sequential scintigraphy (lower) after i.v. injection of ^{131}I-fenetylline in the dog (0–60 min).

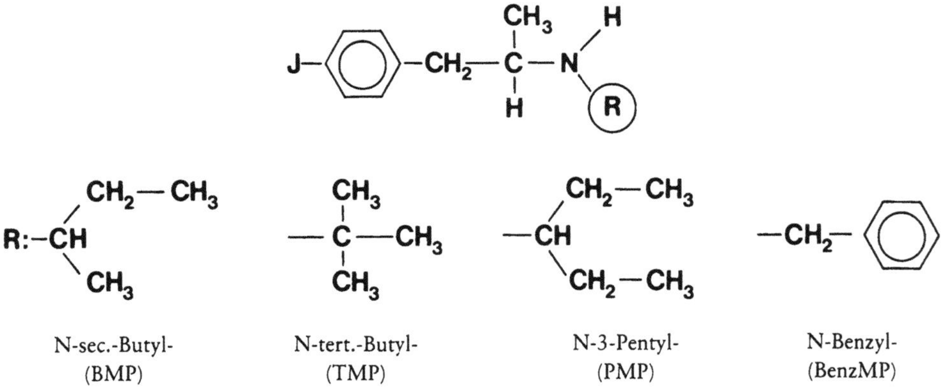

Fig. 3 N-alkyl-derivatives of p-iodoamphetamine.

The names of these compounds are:

- N-(sec.-butyl)-p-iodoamphetamine,
- N-(tert.-butyl)-p-iodoamphetamine
- N-(3-pentyl)-p-iodoamphetamine,

and

- N-(benzyl)-p-iodoamphetamine,

which will be abbreviated BMP, TMP, PMP, BenzMP respectively.

The chemical syntheses of these compounds are shown in fig. 4.

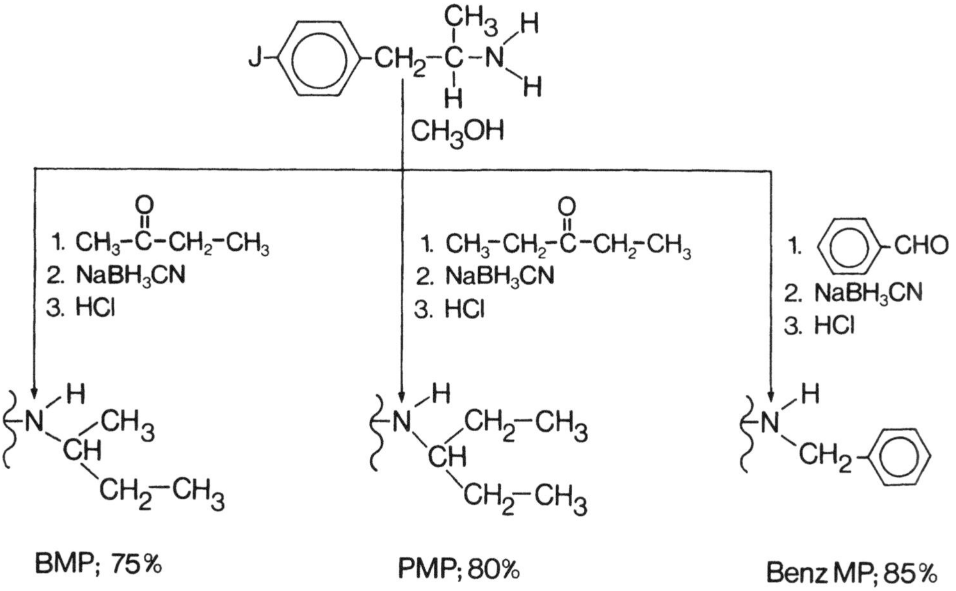

Fig. 4 Chemical syntheses of BMP, PMP and BenzMP.

P-iodoamphetamine was used as starting material, which was, together with the appropriate ketones: Methyl-ethylketone, 3-Pentanone and in the case of BenzMP with Benzaldehyde, stirred at room-temperature for 3–4 hours in the presence of $NaBH_3CN$ in Methanol. Afterwards, the resulting amines were transformed with HCl into the corresponding hydrochlorides and purified by crystallization. The overall-yields were 75%, 80% and 85%.

N-(tert.-butyl)-p-iodoamphetamine, TMP, which cannot be synthesized according to the reaction shown in fig. 4, was produced as demonstrated in fig. 5.

Ter.-butylamine and p-iodobenzylmethylketone were transformed into the desired TMP in a Leuckart-reaction in the presence of formic acid. This TMP was isolated as hydrochloride in an overall-yield of 40%.

The labelling of 4-alkyl-p-iodoamphetamine with ^{131}I is illustrated in fig. 6.

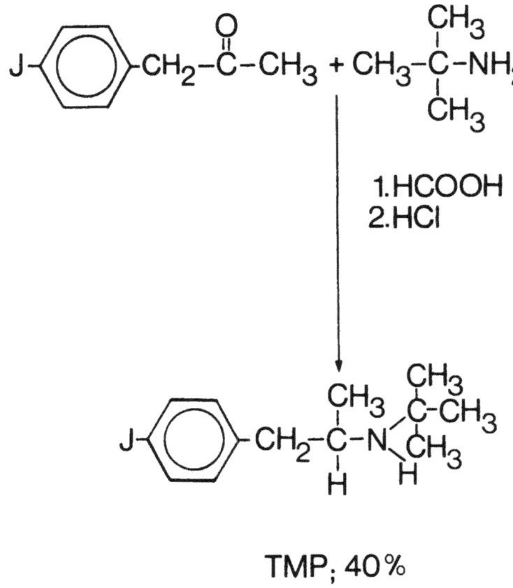

Fig. 5 Chemical synthesis of TMP.

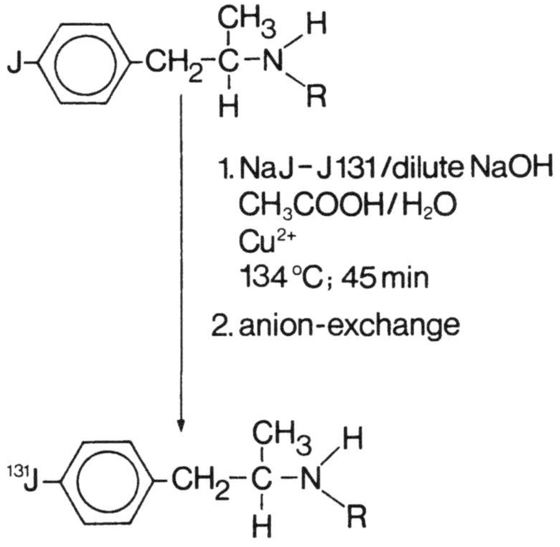

Fig. 6 Labelling method for Alkyl-p-iodoamphetamines.

The respective alkyl-amphetamine is transformed at 134° C for 45 min in aqueous, acetic solution with the required quantity of NaI.^{131}I (in dilute sodium hydroxyde). Still existing free iodine is separated by anion exchange.

By this procedure the amphetamine derivatives were isolated in a radiochemical yield of 90% after purification and sterilfiltration. The specific activity at calibration was in the range of 0.5–1.0 mCi/mg.

The *organ kinetics* of these potential tracers for brain imaging were subsequently determined in animal experiments.

The dog was the first animal used for general evaluation of the organ kinetics of all the respective tracers. Sequential camera scintigraphy following i.v. injection of 500 µCi ^{131}I-labelled compounds revealed cerebral uptake of the afore-mentioned amphetamines.

Fig. 7 shows the time-activity-curve of brain and background 0–60 min after i.v. injection of ^{131}I BMP.

a 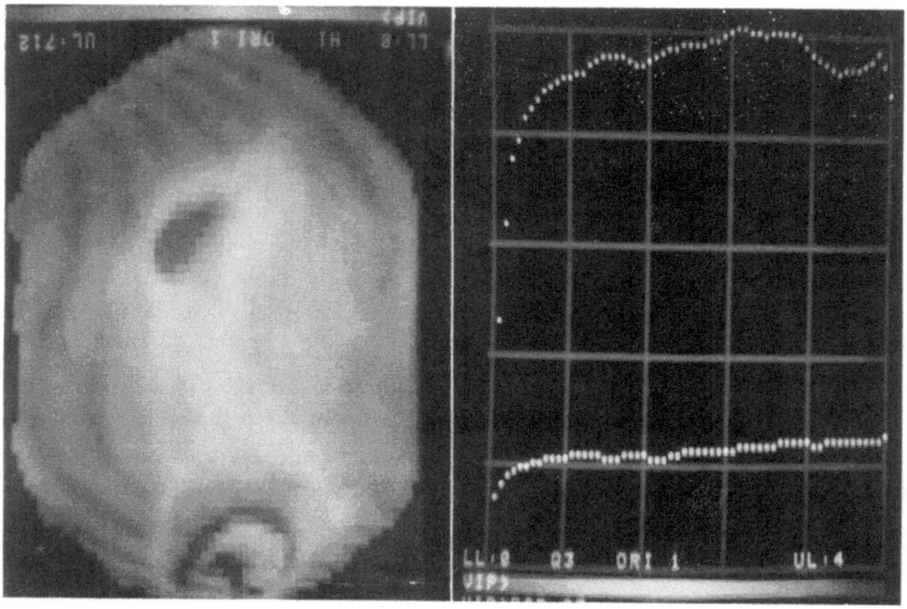 b

Fig. 7 a) sec. butyl amphet.; b) Brain.

The rapid uptake of activity into the brain is demonstrated. The time-activity-curve becomes saturated after about 30 min. The background curve shows a further slight activity increase after this point of time.

The second experimental series consisted of wistar rats weighing 180–200 g: 5 to 10 µCi ^{131}I-labelled BMP, TMP, PMP and BenzMP were administered intravenously. The animals were sacrified 10, 15, 30, 60 and 120 min p.i. and the radioactivity content of tissue specims (brain, cerebellum, liver, lung, spleen, kidney, myocardium, muscle) as well as that in urine and blood samples were measured in a well counter (% dose/g tissue). The most important data of this series are summarized in table 2.

BMP showed the highest brain uptake (1.9%/g) after 30 min, followed by TMP (1.2%/g). PMP and BenzMP did not show such high cerebral accumulation.

A comparison of lung and liver kinetics of IMP and BMP (tab. 3) reveals BMP to have a pulmonary retention much less than that of IMP. The maximum lung activity between 10 and 30 min is 14 and 18% respectively.

Table 2 Concentration of amphetamine derivatives in the brain of rats (n = 5 for each group) (% I131/g tissue)

Derivatives	10′	15′	30′	60′	120′
BMP	1.0	1.2	1.9	0.7	1.0
TMP	0.9	1.0	1.3	1.3	0.9
PMP	0.6	0.9	1.0	1.1	0.7
BenzMP	–	1.1	0.9	1.1	–

Table 3 Lung and liver kinetic of BMP and IMP (% dose/g tissue)

	10′		15′		30′		60′		120′	
	IMP	BMP	IMP	BMP	IMP	BMP	IMP	BMP	IMP	BMP
Lung	31.8	14.0	14.1	7.6	5.3	18.1	10.5	3.4	11.7	6.4
Liver	2.5	1.1	2.9	1.6	1.5	3.5	1.7	1.6	3.5	0.7

The peak liver uptake of BMP is 3.5% after 30 min, followed by a fast decrease to 0.7%/g at 2 hours; IMP having 3.5%/g at 2 hours. With respect to extracerebral radiation burden BMP seems to be superior to IMP.

In the third series of experiments 4 mCi of ^{123}I-labelled BMP as injected in a baboon (15 kg). The specific activity of the ^{123}I-BMP was 1.0 mCi/mg and the iodine ^{124}I content was 1.7% at calibration.

By means of an arterial catheter blood-samples were taken every 5 min from 0–60 min. 60 min p. i. ECT with a rotating gamma-camera was performed. The corresponding results can be defined as follows:

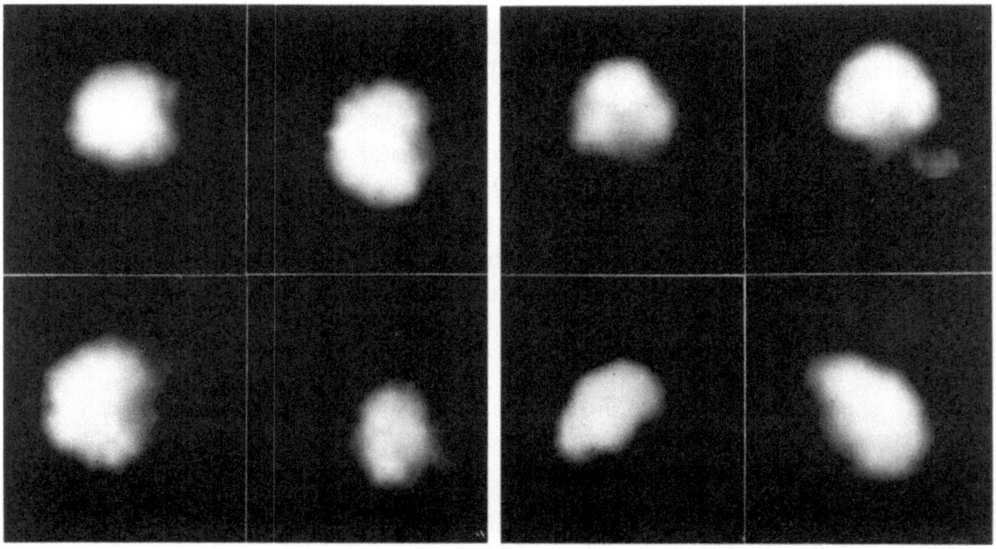

a b c

Fig. 8 a) Baboon (transv.); b) Baboon (coron.); c) Baboon (sagitt.).

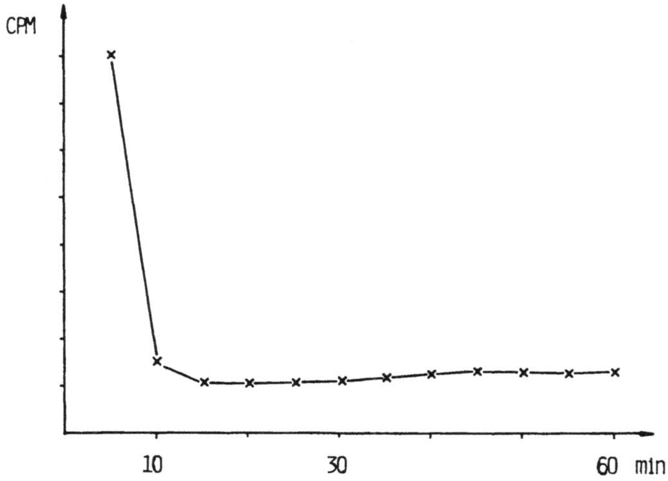

Fig. 9 Time-activity curve of the arterial blood (baboon) after i.v. injection of ^{123}I-BMP.

The transverse, coronal, saggital cuts produced with the help of SPECT, produce pictures with high resolution (fig. 8).

The radioactivity curve in arterial blood (fig. 9) decreases after about 15 min to a minimum and afterwards increases again slightly but continuously up to about 40 min.

From our experimental studies BMP appears at the moment to be the tracer of choice for functional brain imaging based on the following reasons: First, its brain uptake is slightly higher than that of IMP and second, its radiation burden to the lung and liver is considerably lower than that of IMP.

First clinical results with this new ^{123}I-labelled brain imaging agent, which were performed on 31 patients, proved our assumption to be true.

References

[1] Sargent, T., A. Kalbhen, A. T. Shulgin et al.: J. Nucl. Med. **16** (1975) 243.

[2] Winchell, H. S., R. M. Baldwin, T. H. Lin: J. Nucl Med. **21** (1980) 940.
Winchell, H. S., W. D. Horst, L. Braun et al.: J. Nucl. Med. **21** (1980) 947.

[3] Lafrance, N. D., H. N. Wagner, P. Whitehouse et al.: J. Nucl. Med. **22** (1981) 1081.

[4] Hill, T. C., B. L. Holman, R. Lovett et al.: J. Nucl. Med. **23** (1982) 191.
Holman, B. L., T. C. Hill. P. L. Magistretti: Invest. Radiol. **17** (1982) 206.

[5] Biersack, H. J., W. Fröscher, H. Klünenberg et al.: Nuc. Compact. **14** (1983) 62.

[6] Biersack, H. J., A. Hartmann, W. Fröscher et al.: Radioaktive Isotope in Klinik und Forschung, hrsg. v. R. Höfer und H. Bergmann, Verlag Egermann, Wien, Bd. **16** (1984) 11.

[7] Biersack, H. J.: 4th Europ. Symp. on Radiopharmacology, Athens/Greece, Abstract p. 8, March 1984.

[8] Ell, P. J., I. Cullum, M. Donaghy et al.: Lancet 1348 (1984).

[9] Hill, T. C., B. L. Holman, R. Lovett et al.: J. Nucl. Med. **23** (1982) 191.

[10] Holman, B. L., T. C. Hill, P. L. Magistretti: Invest. Radiol. **17** (1982) 206.
[11] Kuhl, D. E., J. R. Barrio, S. C. Huang: Proc. III. World Congr. Nucl. Med. & Biol, ed. by C. Raynaud, Pergamon Press, p. 1731, 1982.
[12] Magistretti, P., R. Uren, D. Shomer: Proc. III. World Congr. Nucl. Med. & Biol., ed. by C. Raynaud, Pergamon Press, p. 139, 1982.
[13] Moretti, J. L., S. Askienazy, C. Raynaud et al.: Proc. III. World Cong., Nucl. Med. & Biol., ed. by C. Raynaud, Pergamon Press, p. 135, 1982.
[14] Podreka, I., K. Höll, P. Dal-Bianco et al.: Radioaktive Isotope in Klinik und Forschung, hrsg. v. R. Höfer und H. Bergmann, Verlag Egermann, Wien, Bd. **16** (1984) 3.
[15] Kung, H. F., K. M. Tramposch, M. Blau: J. Nucl. Med. **24** (1982) 66.
[16] Biersack, H. J., L. Zschachlitz, H. Klünenberg et al.: Nuc. Compact. **15** (1984) 13–18.

Biokinetics of N-Isopropyl,p-^{123}I-Iodoamphetamine in the Human

A. Bischof-Delaloye, B. Delaloye

Recently the investigation of cerebral blood flow with radioactive amines and single photon emission tomography has been more and more widely accepted especially in patients with cerebrovascular disease. These tracers are distributed in the brain proportional to cerebral blood flow. They are lipophilic and – crossing the blood-brain barrier – are extracted almost completely during a single passage through cerebral circulation [1–5]. It seemed us important to know the approximate amount of the injected dose accumulating in brain and other organs, the rapidity of uptake as well as the time of steady state.

Patients and method

For ethical reasons the measurements were performed on patients with minor cerebrovascular disease, brain metastases and focal epilepsy in the interictal state and not on normals. The details of the method are described elsewhere [6a,b], only the most important features will be summarized here. All patients were examined after overnight fasting so that blood volume and cardiac output could be assumed baseline. During 10 minutes before and after injection of the tracer (N-isopropyl-p-iodoamphetamine* labeled with ^{123}I prepared from the ^{127}I (p,5n) ^{123}Xe reaction** – 5 mCi) through an indwelling catheter the patient was allowed to rest in a dark and quiet room, the eyes closed so that external stimuli were kept to a minimum. In fact, after visual or auditory stimulation own and other [7] studies have shown a predominant tracer accumulation in the visual or auditory cortex.

The plasma disappearance of the tracer was followed during the 2 hours after injection of IMP.

Whole body distribution of the tracer was studied with a dual head scintillation camera between 30 and 90 minutes after injection in 11 patients, three of them were restudied 24 and even 48 hours, (2 patients).

* Roche
** EIR

Regions of interest were drawn over brain, lungs, liver/spleen, thyroid and bladder on the anterior and the posterior view. Anterior and posterior counts were averaged and expressed as percent of whole body activity.

Emission single photon tomography of the brain was carried out with a rotating dual head scintillation camera device at several time interval (60 and 120 minutes more recently 14, 45 minutes and 5 hours) following tracer injection. 30 projections per camera head were enregistered at an angular increment of 6 degrees and a counting time of 40–50 seconds per angle. When three-phase studies were performed total rotation was 15 minutes at each sequence (30 seconds per view). 40'000 to 50'000 counts were collected per view that means a total of 3'000'000 counts. Tomographic reconstruction was done with a PDP 11/44 computer equipped with an array processor. Total reconstruction time was 3 to 5 minutes with a slice thickness of 12 mm in a 64 × 64 matrix.

Results

The plasma disappearance curve showed an initial rapid decrease followed by a plateau or a slight increase. The downslope was bi-exponential, the average T ½ being 5 (77%) respectively 60 (23%) minutes.

The organ distribution of activity expressed as percent of the remaining whole body activity is shown on tables 1 to 3.

Table 1 Brain activity in percent of whole body activity at different time intervals after injection of IMP

Time	n	Activity (x ± SE)
30'	11	5.63 ± 0.27
90'	10	6.30 ± 0.28
24 h	3	4.54 ± 0.52
48 h	2	4.48 ± 0.63

Brain activity did slightly but not significantly increase between 30 and 90 minutes after injection. The intracerebral distribution of activity did not change significantly during this time interval. Fig. 1 shows transverse sections of the brain of a patient at the level of the basal ganglia at 1 and 2 hours after injection. The distribution of activity did not change significantly during this time interval.

When tomographic imaging was performed later than two hours post injection evident or discrete changes of intracerebral distribution could be observed.

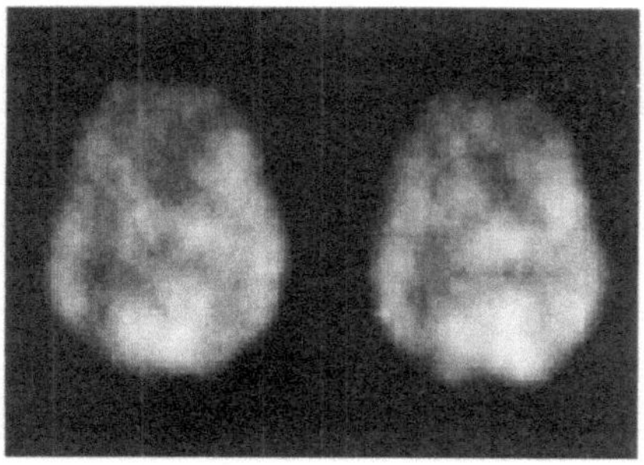

Fig. 1 Transverse sections at the same level in the same patient 60 (left) and 120 minutes (right) after injection of ^{123}I-IMP: no significant difference in tracer distribution can be noticed.

Fig. 2 shows the intracerebral distribution of radioactivity in a patient with reversible ischemic neurological disease at 15, 45 minutes and 5 hours after injection of IMP. The overall activity increased with time (the ECT was performed with an identical time pre-set). The relative hypoactivity of the left middle cerebral artery region is most evident on the early picture on the left, especially in what concerns the left basal ganglia. This relative hypoactivity remains visible at 45 minutes but disappears on the 5 hours picture. In contrary, this picture on the right shows a certain predominance of accumulation in the left basal ganglia.

The pathophysiological substrate to this phenomenon which has been observed by others [11] is unknown up to now. The chemical nature of the labeled compound which passes the blood brain barrier in a delayed manner is also ignored. Table 2 shows that a significant amount of activity leaves the lungs between 30 and 90 minutes after injection. The activitiy lost by the lungs mainly shifts to the liver. This seems probably related to some metabolic processes.

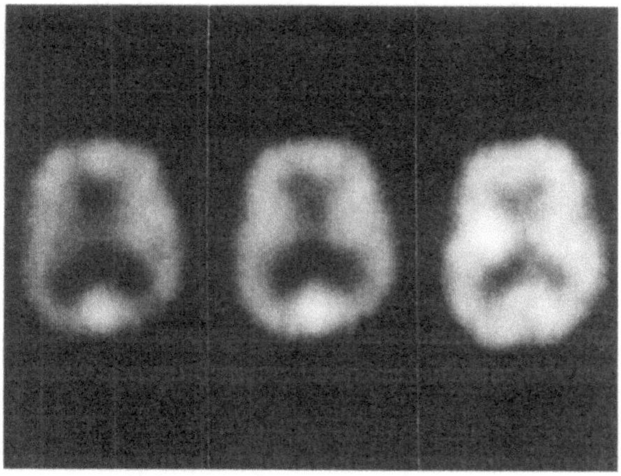

Fig. 2 Transverse sections at the same level in patient with reversible ischemic neurological disease at 15 (left), 45 minutes (middle) and 5 hours (right): the hypoactivity of the left middle cerebral artery region is most striking on the very early image but remains visible at 45′. At 5 hours activity preveals in the left hemisphere especially with respect to the basal ganglia.

Table 2 Lung and liver/spleen activity in percent of whole body activity at different time intervals after injection of IMP

Time	n	Activity (mean ± SE) lungs	liver/spleen
30′	11	30.71 ± 1.96	19.63 ± 0.73
90′	10	24.65 ± 2.06*	22.69 ± 0.76*
24 h	3	25.02 ± 3.76	20.41 ± 1.36*
48 h	2	16.69 ± 4.61	26.57 ± 1.71

* Bartletts significance level

Table 3 Thyroid and bladder activity in percent of whole body activity at different time intervals after injection of IMP

Time	n	Activity (mean ± SE) thyroid	bladder
30′	11	1.03 ± 0.09	0.99 ± 0.36
90′	10	1.11 ± 0.09	2.29 ± 0.38
24 h	3	0.51 ± 0.18	1.47 ± 0.69
48 h	2	0.49 ± 0.22	1.89 ± 1.20

During the following hours activity distribution remains quite stable, nearly no elimination takes place which is not only demonstrated by very low bladder count rates (tab. 3) but also by direct measurements on the 72 hours urinary excretion in two patients which proved to be 6 respectively 8 percent of the injected activity.

We did not observe a significant amount of iodine in the thyroid in these patients but all of them had received contrast medium at the occasion of brain CT examination up to 4 weeks before the IMP study, so that some blocking of the thyroid may be assumed.

Contrary to the observations made in the primate [8] eye activity did not exceed background counts at any moment of the study in particular not on the delayed (24 and 48 h) images, neither on planar nor on tomographic views. This was confirmed by Holman et al. [9].

Discussion

Only a small amount (6–7%) of the injected tracer is extracted and accumulated in the brain, whereas about half of the injected activity is found in lungs and liver.

According to the present data not only brain uptake but also intracerebral distribution may be considered stable between 30 and 90 (120) minutes after injection of

IMP. This stability of uptake and distribution has also been observed by Holman et al. first in the primate [8] and later on in the human [9]. The relative stability of brain activity allows the recording of high count rate tomographic data in spite of the low absolute tracer accumulation in the brain but does not permit to follow rapidly changing phenomena such as effects of pharmaceuticals for instance.

If cerebrovascular abnormalities are to be investigated a very early scan seems to be useful as differences of uptake are more pronounced before reaching equilibrium (fig. 2). This has also been shown by other authors [10, 11] who compared the ^{133}Xe dynamic SPECT with ^{123}I-amphetamine SPECT of the brain. The best correlation between these two methods was obtained with early registration (during the first 10 minutes [10], between 13 and 27 minutes [11]) of IMP brain distribution. These authors [11] also showed the differences of early and late (several hours) intracerebral distribution of activity, which may be very important. Cold areas on the early scan may completely disappear or even become hot on late images (fig. 2). Further investigations are necessary to elucidate this phenomenon especially in what concerns the chemical nature of the labeled compound which passes the blood-brain barrier in a delayed manner, the role of the lungs as a transitory reservoir of this or any other compound and finally the signification in terms of cerebral pathophysiology. If it is easy to imagine that completely destroyed areas of the brain appear as cold regions on early and late IMP scans, it is much more difficult to explain the behaviour of initially cold areas which may become iso- or even hyperactive with respect to normal brain on the delayed images. We have observed this type of early/late distribution patterns more often in patients with transitory cerebrovascular events than in patients with complete stroke. Thus sequential SPECT with labeled amines might perhaps be able to specify further diagnostic and prognostic aspects of cerebrovascular disease. It has to be, however, investigated further how these differences are related to concomitant lung disease. Pistolesi et al. [122] showed a prolonged persistence of HIDPM [13], the other ^{123}I labeled amine currently used for cerebral perfusion studies, within the lungs of patients with probable pulmonary endothelial damage (smokers) and patients with adult respiratory distress syndrome (ARDS).

Conclusion

In spite of the relatively low absolute uptake of ^{123}I-IMP by the brain the distribution of the compound can be studied reliably under steady state conditions between 30 and at least 90 minutes after injection by emission computed tomography.

Even if IMP is distributed to and within the brain according to blood flow there is no doubt that other phenomena than flow and probably also other labeled compounds than IMP itself (metabolites) play a role in the final scintigraphic appearance of the brain in the early and probably much more the late phase after injection. A great amount of work remains still to be done in order to define at least the most important among them but sequential ECT might possibly be able to specify further diagnostic and prognostic aspects of especially ischemic brain disease.

References

[1] Winchell, H. S., R. M. Baldwin, T. H. Lin: Development of ^{123}I-labeled amines for brain studies: Localization of ^{123}I-iodophenylalkylamines in rat brain. J. Nucl. Med. **21** (1980) 940–946.

[2] Winchell, H. S., W. D. Horst, L. Braun: N-Isopropyl-[^{123}]I-p-iodoamphetamine: Single-pass brain uptake and washout; binding to brain synaptosomes; and localization in dog and monkey brain. J. Nucl. Med. **21** (1980) 947–952.

[3] Hill, T. C., B. L. Holman, R. Lovett: Initial experience with SPECT (Single Photon Computerized Tomography) of the brain using N-isopropyl-^{123}I-iodoamphetamine: Concise Communication. J. Nucl. Med. **23** (1982) 191–195.

[4] Holman, B. L., T. C. Hill, P. L. Magistretti: Brain imaging with emission computed tomography and radiolabeled amines. Invest. Radiol. **17** (1982) 206–215.

[5] Kuhl, D. E., J. R. Barrio, S. C. Huang: Quantifying local cerebral blood flow b N-isopropyl-p-[^{123}I]-iodoamphetamine (IMP) tomography. J. Nucl. Med. **23** (1982) 196–203.

[6a] Delaloye, B., A. Bischof: Delaloye: Biodistribution of ^{123}I Amphetamine: First experience and possible clinical applications. Proceedings of a colloquium held at Würenlingen, Switzerland, Oct. 28, 1983, Editions Roche Basle Switzerland 1984. G. K. V. Schultess, A. Bekier and P. A. Schubiger eds.:

[6b] Bischof-Delaloye, A., J. P. Hungerbühler, F. Regli et al.: ^{123}I-iodoamphetamine: Preliminary results on biokinetics and distribution of cerebral blood flow. In: Höfer und Bergmann (eds.): Radioaktive Isotope in Klinik und Forschung, Bd. 16, Egermann, Wien 1984, S. 27.

[7] Podreka, I., P. Dal-Bianco, B. Mamoli: Clinical usefulness of N-isopropyl p-(^{123}I)-iodoamphetamine brain studies (SPECT). In: V. Schulthess, Bekier and Schubiger (eds.): ^{123}I-amphetamine (Perfusamine ^{TM}), Proceedings of a colloquium held at Würenlingen, Switzerland, October 28, 1983. Editiones (Roche), Basle 1984.

[8] Holman, B. L., R. E. Zimmermann, J. R. Schapiro et al.: Biodistribution and dosimetry of N-isopropyl-p-^{123}I-iodoamphetamine in the primate. J. Nucl. Med. **24** (1983) 922–932.

[9] Holman, B. L., R. G. L. Lee, T. C. Hill et al.: A comparison of two cerebral perfusion tracers, N-isopropyl ^{123}I-p-iodoamphetamine and ^{123}I-HIDPM in the human. J. Nucl. Med. **25** (1984) 25–30.

[10] Lassen, N. A., L. Henriksen, S. Holm et al.: Cerebral blood-flow tomography: ^{133}-Xenon compared with isopropyl-^{123}I-amphetamine-iodine. Concise communication. J. Nucl. Med. **24** (1983) 17–21.

[11] Buell, V., P. Schmiedek, C. M. Kirsch et al.: Interhemispheral ratios of perfusion in ^{123}I-amphetamine SPECT and ^{133}Xe dynamic SPECT. A comparative study in patients with cerebrovascular disease (CVD). In: Schmidt, Vauramo (eds.): Nuklearmedizin, 22. Internationale Jahrestagung der Gesellschaft für Nuklearmedizin – Europa, Helsinki, 13.–17. August 1984, Schattauer, Stuttgart 1984.

[12] Pistolesi, M., M. Miniat, N. Mazzuca et al.: Lung kinetics of radioactive HIPDM: A method to detect lung cellular damage in man. In: Schmidt, Vauramo (eds.): Nuklearmedizin, 22. Internationale Jahrestagung der Gesellschaft für Nuklearmedizin – Europa, Helsinki, 13.–17. August 1984, Schattauer, Stuttgart 1984.

[13] Kung, H. F., K. M. Tramposch, M. Blau: A new brain perfusion imaging agent: [^{123}I]-HIPDM: N,N,N'-trimethyl-N'-[2-hydroxy-3-methyl-5-iodobenzyl]-1,3-Propanediamine. J. Nucl. Med. **24** (1983) 66–72.

^{201}Tl-Diethyldithiocarbamate as an Alternative for ^{123}I-Amphetamine in Brain Imaging with SPECT

J. F. de Bruïne, E. A. van Royen, A. Vyth, J. M. B. V. de Jong, Th. C. Hill, H. Venema, J. B. van der Schoot

Introduction

Highly lipophilic radiopharmaceuticals are needed for assessment of regional Brain Perfusion with Single Photon Emission Computed Tomography.

Winchell [1, 2] developed n-isopropyl-p-^{123}I-iodoamphetamine which has been studied intensively the last few years. In a previous study we described the development of ^{201}Tl-Diethyldithiocarbamate [3]. A pilot study in rats proved its high brain uptake. ^{201}Tl-DDC showed a considerable greater brain uptake than ^{201}Tl-Chloride. The brain uptake in rats of ^{201}Tl-DDC was comparable to ^{123}I-IMP as described in literature [1]. For ^{201}Tl-DDC 2.73% of the injected dose per gram wet tissue was found in the rat brain, while Winchell found 2.14% for ^{123}I-IMP.

In the following we compare the results of the administration of ^{201}Tl-DDC and ^{123}I-IMP in rabbits. We will report on the kinetics of brain and lung uptake, the ratio of binding to gray versus white matter and the distribution of both agents to the main organs of the body. Initial quantitative autoradiogaphic results are presented.

Some of the results obtained in human volunteers with SPECT employing ^{201}Tl-DDC will be demonstrated.

Materials and methods

The synthesis of ^{201}Tl-Diethyldithiocarbamate has been described elsewhere [3]. ^{123}I-IMP was obtained from "Cygne" (Technische Hogeschool Eindhoven, Netherlands). The ^{123}I is cyclotron produced and contaminated with less than 2.5% ^{124}I at calibration time. The radiochemical purity is more than 99% while the specific activity is more than 50 Ci/gram ^{123}I-IMP.

A General Electric Maxi Camera 400 autotune ZS with a lower energy general purpose collimator was used for performing dynamic studies. 0.5 mCi ^{201}Tl-DDC (six rabbits) or ^{123}I-IMP (five rabbits) were injected into an ear vein, following anaesthesia with 1–2 ml Hypnorm. Time activity curves were obtained for brain, lungs, liver and kidney after background subtraction.

Between 25 and 45 min after injection of ^{201}Tl-DDC (N = 4) or ^{123}I-IMP (N = 4) eight rabbits were killed with 2–3 ml pentobarbital 10% and thoracotomy for tissue sampling. Brain perfusing was performed with NaCl solution (0.9%) and formaldehyde (4%). Organs were removed and weighed. Tissue samples of gray and white matter, basal ganglia, cerebellum, lung, liver and kidney were weighed and counted (Gamma Counter C 64 000/PG 4000). After correction for dose the counts were expressed in percentage of the dose per gram wet tissue.

Two rabbits were killed for macroautoradiography 5 min after injection. One received 1.84 mCi ^{201}Tl-DDC, the other one 2.46 mCi ^{123}I-IMP. After perfusion the brain was frozen and cut into 20 micron sections. The sections were placed on film (Agfa Osray M3). Digital images were made with a special computer adapted microdensitometer 3CS (Joyce/Laebel). Regions of interest were delineated with a light pen and after background subtraction cortical gray/white matter and cortical gray matter/basal ganglia ratios were defined.

Human studies: After the injection of 3 mCi of ^{201}Tl-DDC in a human volunteer planar images of the head were obtained, as well as the whole body on a gamma camera. A SPECT study was acquired with the Harvard multidetector brain system.

Results

In fig. 1 time activity curves for brain and lungs are shown. The peak value for ^{123}I-IMP in the lung is reached at 1 min after injection, whereafter the activity falls down to 30% of maximum at 18 min. The maximum level for ^{201}Tl-DDC in the lung is reached at 0.5 min, whereafter there is a very quick decrease of the activity and the 30% of maximum level is found at 2 min after injection. For both radiopharmaceuticals there is a rapid increase in activity in the brain, which is significantly faster for ^{201}Tl-DDC as shown in fig. 2. The brain activity for ^{201}Tl-DDC remains fairly constant after 1.5 min, and for ^{123}I-IMP after 3.5 min.

The tissue sampling results are demonstrated in tab. 1. For both radiopharmaceuticals there is an almost equal percentage brain uptake of the dose: 1.46 for ^{201}Tl-DDC and 1.14 for ^{123}I-IMP. The gray/white matter ratio found by sampling proved to be also equal: 1.44 ± 0.18 S.E.M. for ^{201}Tl-DDC and 1.14 ± 0.07 S.E.M. for ^{123}I-IMP. Lung activity at time of killing of the rabbits differs remarkable: 0.53% of the ^{201}Tl-DDC dose versus 8.32% of the ^{123}I-IMP dose. Liver and kidney results are also shown in tab. 1.

The digital autoradiographic images of the brain sections are shown in fig. 3 and 4. For both radiopharmaceuticals clear demarcation of gray and white matter is seen. The quantitative results are demonstrated in tab. 2 and are eqal for both.

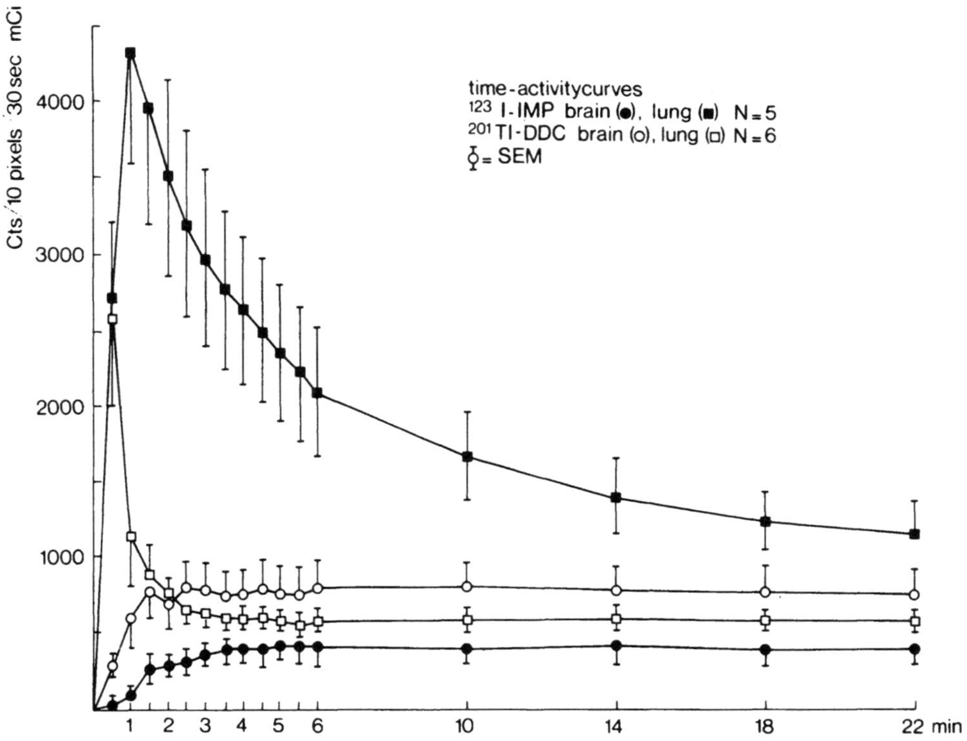

Fig. 1 I^{123}–IMP and ^{201}Tl–DDC time-activity curves for lung and brain.

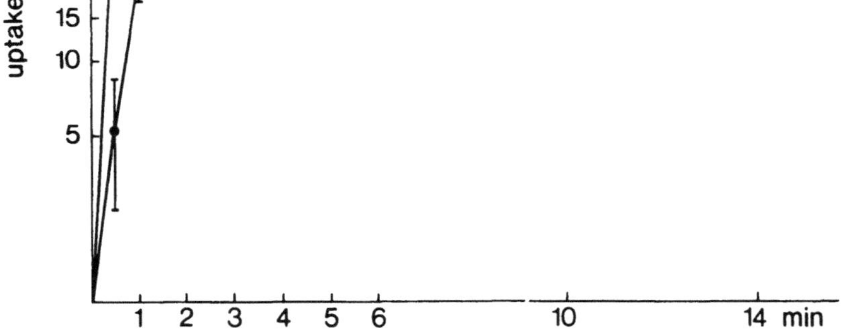

Fig. 2 Brain time activity curves for ^{123}I–IMP (●, N=5) and ^{201}Tl–DDC (O, N=6) in rabbits (M±SEM, semilogarithmic scale).

Table 1 Distribution of activity in % of the dose in rabbits killed between 25 and 45 min. after injection

	^{201}Tl-DDC per organ	per gram wet tissue	^{123}I-IMP per organ	per gram wet tissue
brain (total)	1.46 ± 0.28	–	1.14 ± 0.18	–
cerebellum	–	0.18 ± 0.05	–	0.14 ± 0.02
basal ganglia	–	0.16 ± 0.04	–	0.16 ± 0.01
white matter	–	0.12 ± 0.03	–	0.13 ± 0.02
cortical gray matter	–	0.16 ± 0.04	–	0.18 ± 0.02
lungs	0.53 ± 0.17	0.04 ± 0.02	8.32 ± 0.39	0.48 ± 0.11
liver	14.35 ± 1.85	0.09 ± 0.01	8.68 ± 1.12	0.08 ± 0.01
kidneys	5.45 ± 1.18	0.29 ± 0.04	5.06 ± 1.99	0.33 ± 0.05
	n = 4, M ± SEM		n = 4, M ± SEM	

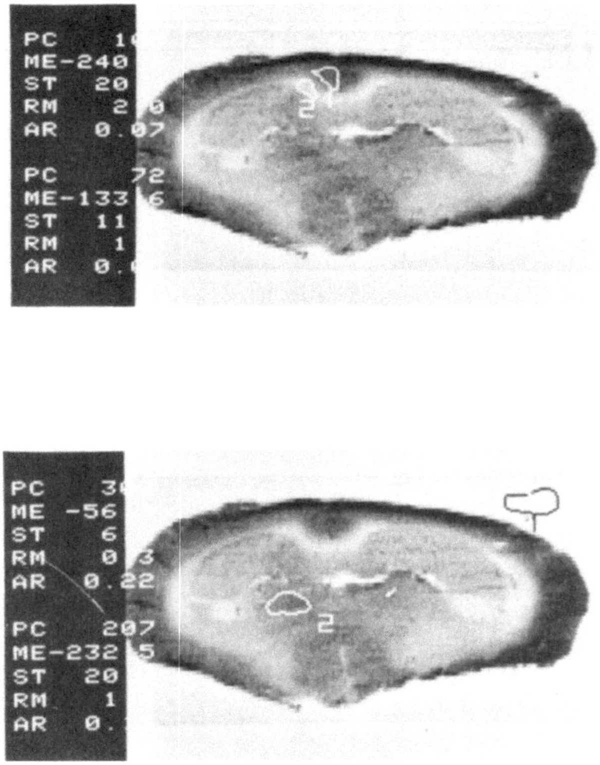

Fig. 3 ^{201}Tl–DDC digital macroautoradiographic images, coronal sections of rabbit brain. Regions of interest are delineated.

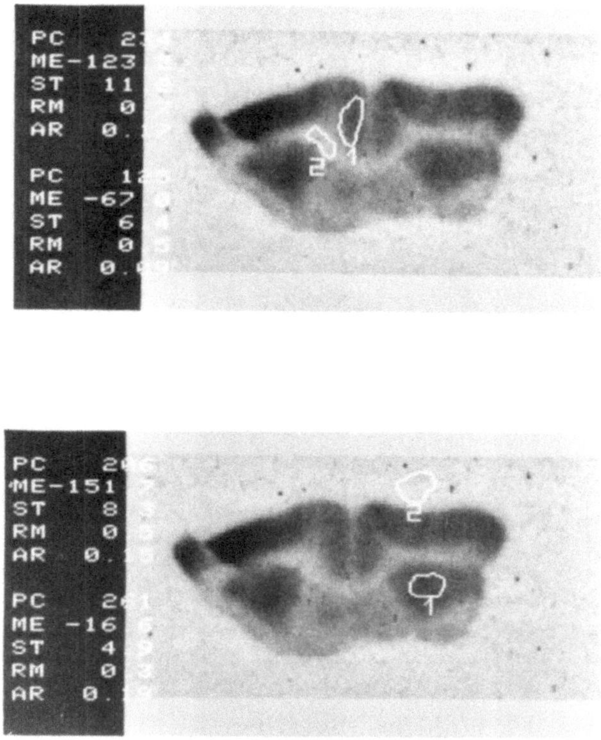

Fig. 4 ^{123}I–IMP digital macroautoradiographic images, coronal sections of rabbit brain. Regions of interest are delineated.

Table 2 Quantitative results of autoradiography

ratio	^{201}Tl-DDC	^{123}I-IMP
cortical gray/white matter	2.4	2.1
cortical gray matter/basal ganglia	1.1	0.8
	N = 1	N = 1

The total body image and the planar images of a human volunteer show about 90 min. after injection a good brain retention (figs. 5 and 6). The tomographic results obtained in an other human volunteer 3 hours after injection of ^{201}Tl-DDC are demonstrated in fig. 7. Gray and white matter contrast fairly and the image resembles to those obtained with ^{123}I-IMP.

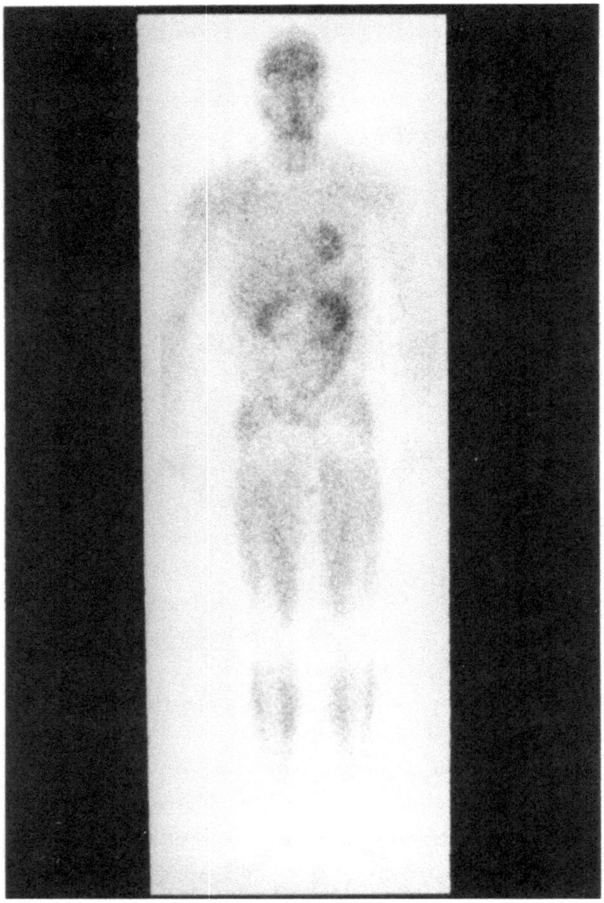

Fig. 5 Total body image about 90 min. after injection of 3 mCi ^{201}Tl–DDC in human volunteer.

Discussion

The results of our study in rabbits with ^{123}I-IMP and ^{201}Tl-DDC show almost similar brain uptake, gray to white matter ratio and macroautoradiographic results. The somewhat slower brain uptake for ^{123}I-IMP relatively to ^{201}Tl-DDC may be explained by its greater lung retention. Although the physical half life time and energy of ^{201}Tl are not ideal, the images obtained in human volunteers are promising. The whole body distribution pattern of ^{201}Tl-DDC is apart from the brain, very similar to the pattern of ^{201}Tl-chloride. The radiation dose of ^{201}Tl-DDC, although higher than for ^{123}I-amphetamine, is comparable to the dose administered in ^{201}TI cardiac studies except for the brain. But more studies have to be done on this subject. Advantages of the ^{201}Tl-DDC preparation are good availability at a relatively low cost and a more prompt brain uptake which is important in blood flow studies. The clinical use of ^{201}Tl-DDC SPECT may become of value in studying the early events in cerebral ischaemia in the near future especially due to its 24 h availability.

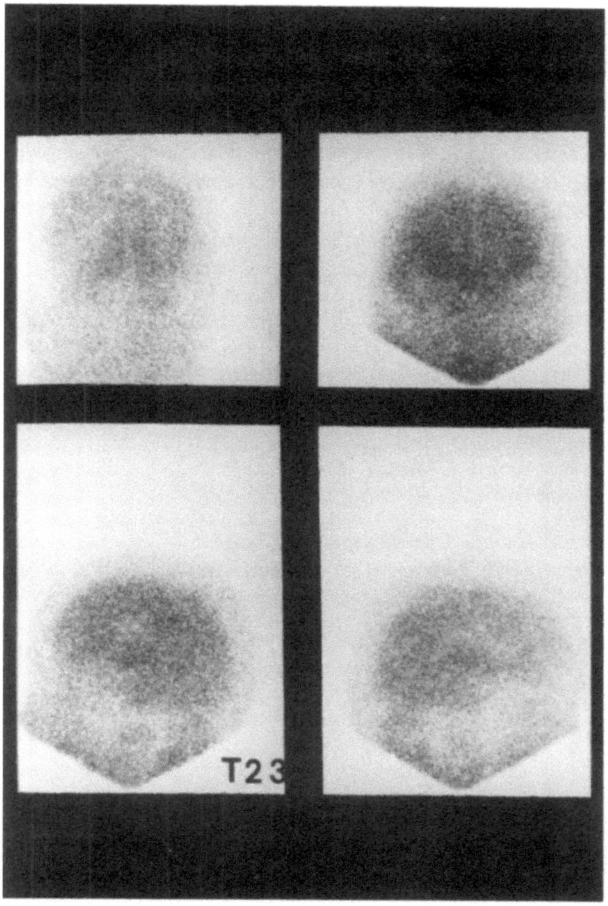

Fig. 6 Planar images about 90 min. after injection of 3 mCi ^{201}Tl–DDC in human volunteer.

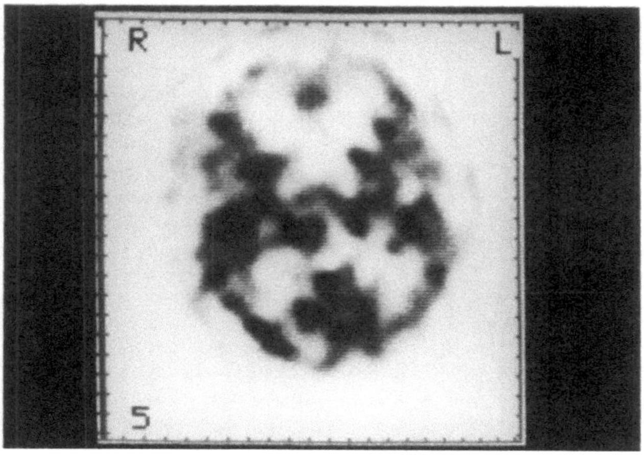

Fig. 7 Axial S.P.E.C.T. image of human brain, 3 hours after injection of 3 mCi ^{201}Tl–DDC.

References

[1] Winchell, H. S., R. M. Baldwin, T. H. Lin: Development of ^{123}I-labelled amines for brain studies: localisation of ^{123}I-iodophenylalkylamines in rat brain. J. Nucl. Med. 21 (1980) 940–946.

[2] Winchell, H. S., W. D. Horst, L. Braun et al.: N-isopropyl-[^{123}I]p-iodoamphetamine: single pass brain uptake and washout: binding to brain synaptosomes, and localisation in dog and monkey brain. J. Nucl. Med. 21 (1980) 947–952.

[3] Vyth, A., P. J. Fennema, J. B. van der Schoot: ^{201}Tl-diethyldithiocarbamate: a possible radiopharmaceutical for brain imaging. Pharm. Weekbl. (Sci.) 5 (1983) 213–216.

Development of a Lipophilic ^{99m}Tc Complex Useful for Brain Perfusion Evaluation with Conventional SPECT Imaging Equipment

R. D. Neirinckx, D. P. Nowotnik, R. D. Pickett, R. C. Harrison, P. J. Ell

The need for measurement of brain perfusion

The advent of computerized tomography brought the possibility of diagnosing morphological abnormalities in brain, as in other organs, in such fine detail that the technique replaced the old radionuclide test of the blood brain barrier (BBB) integrity virtually completely. Thus, it became possible to define the size and location of tumours and infarcted areas very accurately. But, it also became clear that the detection of brain abnormalities through the identification of morphological changes only established the course for treatment of afflictions such as stroke at a stage when much of the damage was already irreversible. The primary determinant of haemodynamic disturbances, i. e. the cerebral blood flow, can only be determined by CT through the use of contrast agents, an unpleasant and potentially dangerous procedure.

The assessment of brain perfusion rather than morphology represents a tool to the clinician with which he can predict the onset of neurological problems before they reach the catastrophic proportions that lead to morphologic changes. Anthough knowledge of regional blood-flow through the brain does not necessarily reflect the tissue's metabolic condition, changes in its value can be symptomatic of developing disease before morphologic changes take place. Changes in blood flow are apparent immediately after the onset of stroke symptoms and most dementias may lead to changes in blood flow. Unequivocal identification of dementias can be done by performing a biopsy, but this is clearly an undesirable process.

Desired properties of a radioactive compound for rCBF evaluation

In experimental animal work it has been shown that regional blood flow can be measured by quantitation of the deposition by capillary blockade of microspheres of appropriate size. The technique has been used as a standard against which to measure the capability of other compounds to measure rCBF.

For clinical diagnosis one can consider the use of a "chemical microsphere", i. e. a compound which will be completely retained in the brain without having to revert to capillary blockade. This can be accomplished by ensuring passage of the chemical through the BBB and retention in the brain tissue. Through measurement of a radioactive isotope, tagged to the "chemical microsphere" one can evaluate rCBF. To achieve uptake in brain, the chemical microsphere must first cross the intact BBB. This can be accomplished by active transport, facilitated diffusion or passive diffusion.

Active transport and facilitated diffusion are very structure-sensitive mechanisms, since they involve binding to protein carrier-molecules. The rate of passive diffusion depends on the size, charge and lipophilicity of the molecule. Small hydrophobic molecules such as O_2, Xe and benzene and small uncharged polar molecules such as H_2O, CO_2 and glycerol cross the lipid bilayer readily. Ions such as H^+ or Na^+ and large uncharged polar molecules are virtually excluded. For example, the permeability by passive diffusion of the cell membrane lipid bilayer for H_2O and K^+ differ by a factor 10^{10}.

The choice of the radioactive isotope used to label lipophilic molecules influences the properties of the molecule's permeability through the BBB. Molecules that can cross the BBB can preserve that capability when labelled with ^{11}C, ^{13}N, ^{15}O or even ^{18}F, and highly extracted compounds labelled with these isotopes can thus be used to evaluate rCBF. However, the practicability of these isotopes is very limited, whereas most isotopes that do have attractive nuclear characteristics are isotopes of elements that are not normally part of molecules that cross the BBB. This leads to compounds that are not normally present in a biological system and virtually eliminates the possibility that such compounds will be actively transported through the BBB. When non-biological labels are used for measurement of rCBF one is practically limited to the use of small lipophilic agents. Whereas a microsphere resides permanently in the capillary bed of the brain the "chemical microspheres" that cross the BBB have widely differing brain clearance characteristics. Agents that remain unchanged in the brain such as $^{15}O\text{-}H_2O$ or Xenon wash quickly out of the brain, whereas those undergoing change may be inhibited from washing out of the brain tissue. The residence time required for imaging of the radioactive compound in the brain is dependent upon the detection mode employed. To allow adequate time for most detection systems to carry out a study it is necessary for the compound to be retained for a finite time. In practical terms the rotating gamma camera is the preferred instrument, because it is a versatile low cost system. However, a typical tomographic study with the rotating gamma camera takes about 20–30 minutes, during which time the activity distribution in the brain may be allowed to change only minimally. Thus, the requirements for a radiopharmaceutical that can measure rCBF can be summarized as:

1. The compound should be neutral and lipophilic for passive diffusion, or otherwise actively transported through the BBB.
2. The extraction efficiency of the compound into the brain must be high.

3. The distribution of the compound must be proportional to blood flow, i.e. it should not redistribute in the brain after the initial deposition.
4. The compound should clear only slowly from brain.
5. The radioisotope used should be coninuously available, so as to make diagnosis with the radiopharmaceutical possible at any time.
6. The compound should be easy and safe to use.
7. The radioisotope should be optimum for use with a gamma-camera.

Choice of radioisotope

The requirement for long retention is the major challenge in the development of a synthetic compound, containing foreign atoms. Such compounds are not normally metabolized, unless the can be made to mimic substrates. Examples are ^{18}F-deoxy glucose and ^{123}I-N-isopropyl amphetamine (IMP). However, these compounds are not readily available. To meet all the requirements, a radioactive rCBF agent should contain the generator produced ^{99m}Tc. Incorporation of that isotope almost certainly restricts the capability of a molecule to cross the BBB to the passive diffusion mechanism, for which a small, lipophilic ^{99m}Tc-complex is most suitable.

Very few ligands are known to carry technetium across the BBB and most work has centered on PnAO, BAT and DTS derivatives [1, 2, 3] (fig. 1). Whereas these backbone ligands form lipophilic Tc-complexes that are extracted in brain-tissue, they are not retained and their distribution can only be measured with fast static-ring devices, which are expensive and not yet widely-available. The incorporation of a moiety to elicit trapping of the radioactive complex is thus needed to give the compound wide diagnostic utility.

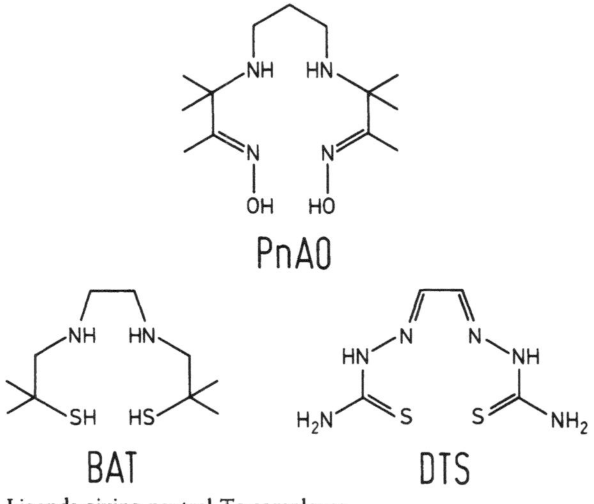

Fig. 1 Ligands giving neutral Tc-complexes.

Choice of trapping mechanism

One approach to the trapping of compounds in the brain entails addition to a known back-bone ligand of a moeity that ensures interaction of the compound with brain-selective mechanisms. For example to explain the trapping of (IMP) [4, 5] interaction with receptors, with monoamine oxidases or with acidic structures inside the brain can be involved. The trapping of PIPSE, MOSE and HIPDM [6] has been explained in terms of a "pH sħift" phenomenon, whoch rests on the higher acidity of the brain as compared to blood. Trapping of ^{201}Tl-DDC [7] could be explained as being caused by an acid-induced decomposition of the DDC-moiety.

The mechanism of trapping of some of the ^{99m}Tc-complexes described in this article can be explained by opening of a weakened hydrogen-bond in the back-bone molecule itself through short-term interaction of the oxime groups of the PAO ligand with molecules that are able to form hydrogen bonds. This short-term intermolecular interaction could trigger an irreversible intra-molecular reaction which renders the ^{99m}Tc complex less lipophilic.

Parameters affecting the permeability of compounds through the blood-brain barrier

The questions we have since tried to answer through evaluation of a series of PAO-derviatives, synthesized at Amersham International were:

(1) How does substitution of the ligand affect the lipophilicity of the complexes?
(2) How does lipophilicity affect the permeability through the BBB?
(3) Is there a Molecular Weight (M. W.) cut-off point beyond which the ^{99m}Tc-complexes do not cross the BBB to an appreciable extent?
(4) How does substitution in the 2- and 8-positions affect the stability of the compound? (fig. 2).

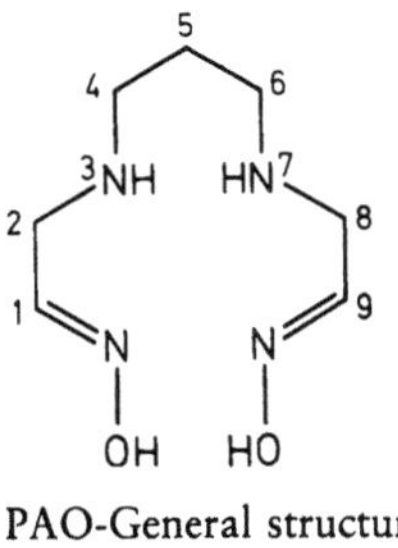

Fig. 2 PAO-General structure and numbering system.

(1) Lipophilicity changes

Propylene amine oxime (PnAO) was shown by Troutner and Volkert to form a neutral, lipophilic technetium complex [1]. The Amersham International laboratories first synthesized a number of alkyl-derivatives of PnAO in order to evaluate the effect of increased alkyl chain length on the lipophilicity of the Tc-complexes. For this purpose, derivatization was carried out at the 1 and 9 position. Lipophilicity was determined by an hplc method, and the results obtained were compared with theoretical lipophilicity values calculated from the experimental ^{99m}Tc-PnAO lipophilicity and the Hansch fragmental constants [8].

*(2) **Permeability of the BBB for ^{99m}Tc-complexes of varying lipophilicity***

The retention in-vivo 2 min after i.v. injection in rats was taken as a measure of relative BBB permeability for the ^{99m}Tc-complexes. Previous dissection work had indicated that even freely diffusible compounds are still largely retained in the brain at that time point.

*(3) **Permeability as a function of M. W.***

There are indications that beyond a maximum M. W. the compound's diffusion through the BBB is severely hindered [9]. In the case of lipophilic ^{99m}Tc-complexes described here whose M. W. differences are solely accomplished through variation of the chain length of the substituting alkyl groups the increasing M. W. parallels increasing lipophilicity and both effects are thus difficult to separate.

*(4) **Variation in compound stability by altering ring-substitution***

We have since sought to vary the stability of the PAO-ring through changes in the substituting alkyl groups on the 2 and 8 position of the molecule. Because of the ring conformation it was assumed that substitution in these positions would most-strongly affect the inter-atomic distance between the oxygen of the oxime-functions and thus affect the complex stability.

Methods

Synthesis of simple alkyl analogues of PnAO

The synthetic scheme is summarized in fig. 3.

The olefin is converted to the corresponding chloronitroso compound by treatment with nitrosylchloride (generated *in-situ* from amylnitrite and concentrated hydrochloric acid). The chloronitroso derivative was isolated by crystallisation. Reaction of chloronitroso derivative with propylenediamine (2:1 ratio of reagents) in refluxing methanol afforded the PAO derivative. During the reaction a proton shift converted the nitrosyl functionality to oxime. The lower homologues were isolated as crystalline solids in the free base form, while the high homologues were obtained as hydrochloride salts. PAO derivatives which contained a single methyl group at the 2- and 8-positions were prepared from 3-chloro-2-butanone oxime, as shown in fig. 3.

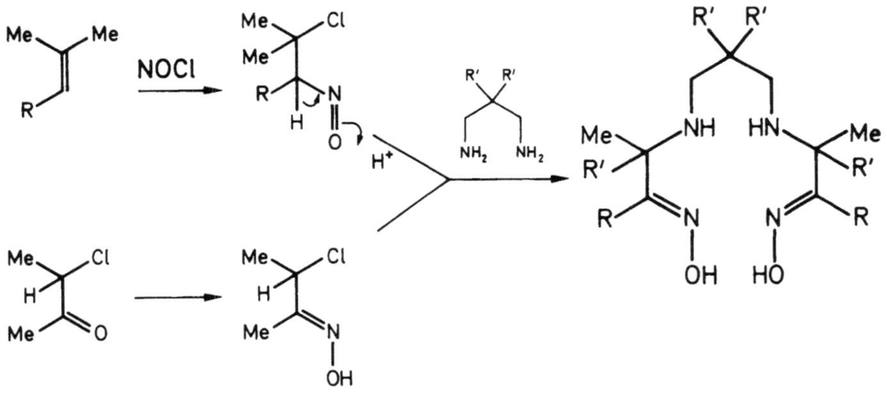

Fig. 3 Synthesis of simple alkyl derivatives of PnAO.

Preparation of the ^{99m}Tc-complexes

The preparation of the ^{99m}Tc-complexes of the various PAO-derivatives followed very similar protocols:

1 mg of the ligand is dissolved in 1 ml ethanol and 0.2 ml of a saturated stannous tartrate solution in isotonic saline is added.

Subsequently 1 ml of ^{99m}Tc pertechnetate is added, followed by 5 ml of N_2-purged isotonic saline.

The radiochemical purity of the ensuing preparation is checked by TLC and reverse-phase HPLC and was always higher than 90 percent 15 min after preparation.

Measurement of protein binding

A sample (100 µl) of the ^{99m}Tc-complex preparation was added to 1 ml human plasma protein (albumin fraction). After 20 minutes at ambient temperature the mixture was transferred to a centrifugal concentrator (Centricon-30, Amicon Core P) and centrifuged to displace a volume not exceeding 110 µl. The radioactivity and volumes of the centrifugate and retentate were measured. The percentage of activity bound was calculated assuming that the activity in the centrifugate was not protein bound and the radioactive concentration of the centrifugate was identical to the radioactive concentration of non protein bound complex in the retentate. Allowance was made for the volume fraction of plasma proteins in the retentate (6% of total volume).

Lipophilicity determination

An HPLC method was used to determine lipophilicity. The technique was based upton the observed similarity between the hydrophilic partitioning process of reverse-phase HPLC and that of traditional octanol-water partitioning.

Several non-radioactive compounds with known octanol-water partition coefficients (P) were selected as standards. The retention time (t) of each was determined using a Hamilton PRP-1 column with an isocratic mixture of THF/0.02M phosphate buffer as eluant, at 25 °C. The capacity factors (K') were calculated according to the formula $K' = (t-t_o)/t_o$ where t_o is the elution time of a non-retained substance ($NaNO_3$). A calibration curve was constructed by plotting log_nK' versus $lop_{10}P$. Retention times were then measured for the ^{99m}Tc-complexes, log_nK' values derived, and $log_{10}P$ values determined using this calibration curve. Each determination was performed in triplicate.

In-vivo evaluation in rats

Sprague-Dawley rats were used throughout the in-vivo evaluation. Animals anaesthetized with uretane were injected with a 0.1 ml solution of the complex in isotonic saline. They were killed at either 2 min or 1 hour after injection and the following organs resected: brain, blood, liver, lungs, heart, kidneys, bladder and muscle. The ^{99m}Tc-activity was counted in an automatic gamma-counter, corrected for decay and expressed as activity/whole organ.

Preliminary clinical data

We have since chosen one of the PAO-derivatives, hexamethyl-PAO (HM-PAO) as the most desirable ligand because of its superior in-vitro and in-vivo characteristics. Freeze-dried batches of the ligand, containing Sn[11] as a reductant for pertechnetate have been manufactured aseptically and their sterility and apyrogenicity verified. Absence of toxicity for dosages up to 890 times the human equivalent has been demonstrated. Product vials were labelled with ^{99m}Tc and up to 20 mCi administered to healthy volunteers. Tomographic images were made between 30′ and 60′ after injection by means of a rotating gamma-camera and whole-body scans were performed up to 4 hours after injection by means of a scanning gamma camera.

Results

Effect of alkyl chain length on lipophilicity

The lipophilicity values obtained by the HPLC method varied linearly with the length of the substituting alkyl chains and were very close to the theoretically calculated values (fig. 4).

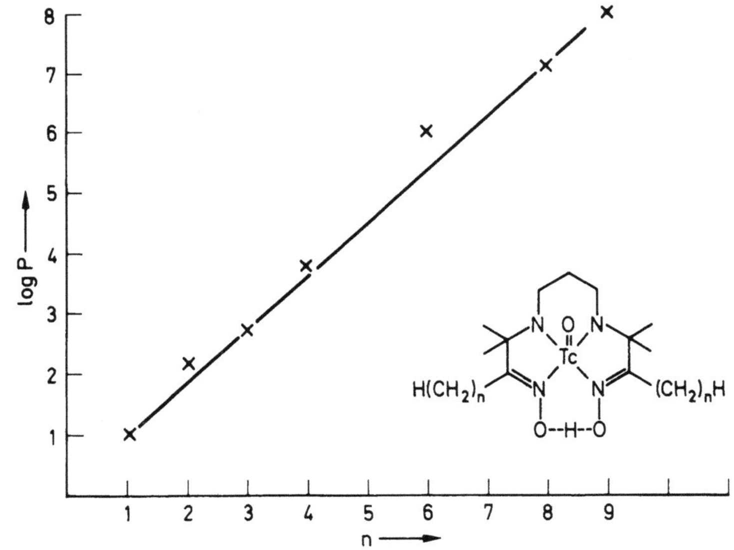

Fig. 4 Graph of log P (determined by hplc) against alkyl chain length.

Effect of lipophilicity on brain uptake in rats

The relationship between $\log_{10}P$ of the ^{99m}Tc-complexes of a series of alkyl-substituted PAO ligands and their relative brain-uptake in rats 2 min after intravenous injection is summarized in fig. 5.

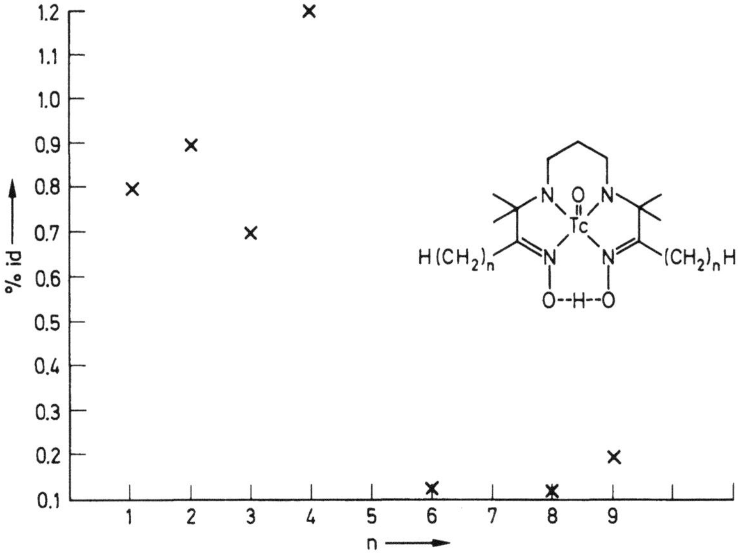

Fig. 5 Graph of brain uptake (%id/whole organ) in rats at 2 min p.i. against alkyl chain length of ^{99m}Tc-PnAO derivatives.

Effect of lipophilicity on protein binding

The relationship between lipophilicity and protein binding for a large number of ^{99m}Tc-complexes of alkyl-derivatized PnAO complexes is summarized in fig. 6.

A rapid increase in protein binding is noticed for compounds with $\log_{10}P$ values ranging between 0.5 and 3.5.

Preliminary clinical results

A whole-body image, obtained 4 hours after injection of a long-retained member of this series is shown in fig. 7.

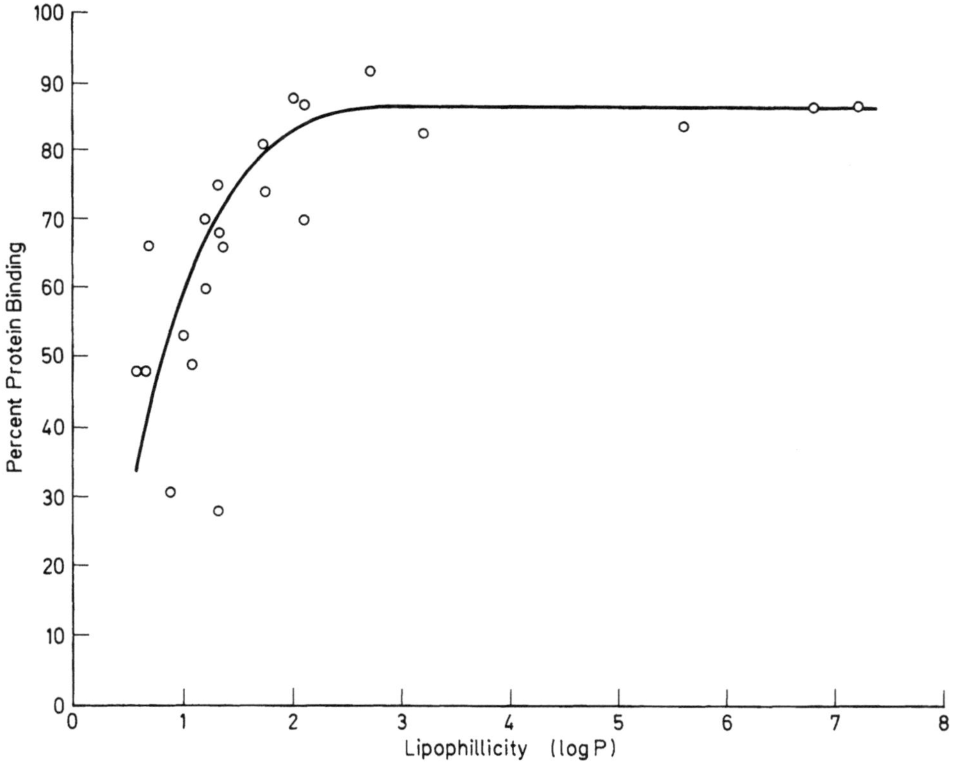

Fig. 6 Protein binding vs. lipophillicity.

Discussion

The relationship found between lipophilicity and brain uptake at 2′ in rats of the ^{99m}Tc-complexes of the PAO analogues is in agreement with the finding of Dischino et al. [10] that the ideal lipophilicity for BBB permeability ranges between log P = 0.9 and 2.5 and that of Hansch et al. [11] that the log P should ideally be 2.0 ± 0.3.

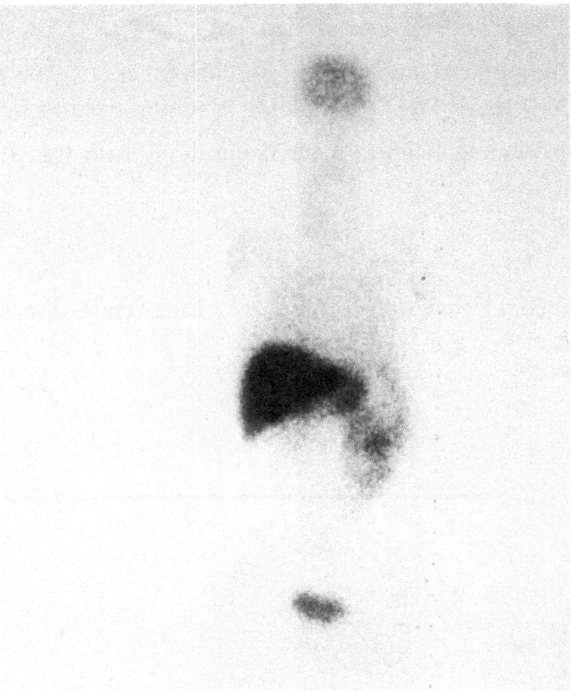

Fig. 7 Clinical results: A whole-body-image.

The fact that the extraction efficiency of alcohols was dropping rapidly for log P >2.5, while the ^{99m}Tc-PAO complexes seem to exhibit the same behaviour for log P >4, may reflect a different degree of protein bindings vs. lipophilicity for these two different classes of compounds.

The permeability of lipid membranes depends not only on the lipophilicity, but also on the molecular weight of the compounds. Levin [8] evaluated the capillary permeability coefficient, P_c, of a series of compounds and compared these with a theoretical value, calculated from the octanol/water partition coefficient, P, and the molecular weight of the compound. The relationship developed by him was:

$$10\text{g } P_c = -4.605 + 0.4115 \log [P(M_r)^{-1'2}]$$

and demonstrates the importance of both M. W. and lipophilicity as determinants of permeability through lipid membranes. He also estimated a M. W. cut-off for significant BBB passage as lying between 400 and 657 Daltons.

Our series of ^{99m}Tc-labelled PAO derivatives confirms the latter statement. The relative brain uptake of these complexes fell very sharply between M. W. 468 and 524, despite an increase in lipophilicity.

In the limited M. W. range which we have studied its effect on brain permeability may well be negligible and the sudden drop-off in brain uptake for the very lipophilic compounds could reflect a very high affinity for blood proteins. Since our measurements were carried out after intra venous injection this protein binding should be taken into account. We found the protein binding to increase dramatically between log P = 0.5 and 3.5 and the sudden BBB permeability deterioration between log P = 4 and 6 might reflect stronger protein binding by such highly-lipophilic compounds.

Most of the suggested trapping mechanisms for brain retention of radioactive compounds involve a reaction of these compounds with brain constituents. The Redox mechanism, receptor binding or monoamine oxidase inhibitors all involve such a potentially dangerous interaction. Many amines, for example, have known physiological effects. Apart from the drawbacks of the ^{123}I used with iodoamphetamine, the compound is being metabolized in the brain, which could have side-effects in the patient. We have elected to use a ^{99m}Tc-labelled agent, whose retention in brain is caused by an intramolecular rearrangement which leads to a drastic change in lipophilicity and thus permeability of the BBB for this compound.

The trapping mechanism of the selected compound is thought to be caused by conversion to a hydrophilic complex, within the brain, possibly by opening of the bond between the oxime groups of the ^{99m}Tc-complex. The hydrogen bonds between the oxime-groups of the complex are inherently weak and probably sensitive to intermolecular hydrogen-bonding molecules which will compete for each oxime-group. By varying the derivatization of the ring, one can alter the strength of the hydrogen bond between them. We have since found that substituent changes at the 2 and 8 position of the ensuing ^{99m}Tc-complex. It is speculated that by weakening the hydrogen bond through substituent changes ist may become more vulnerable to intermolecular interactions with, for example, free ligand molecules or certain proteins. The ensuing ring opening may allow the oxime groups to isomerize to the Z-configuration, which in turn could lead to the formation of a stable bond between the oxime oxygens and the Tc-core of the complex. This would lead to a stable 6 membered ring (fig. 8) and make the isomerisation irreversible. Preliminary data, concerning the effect of ligand concentration on the conversion rate in-vitro tend to confirm this hypothesis.

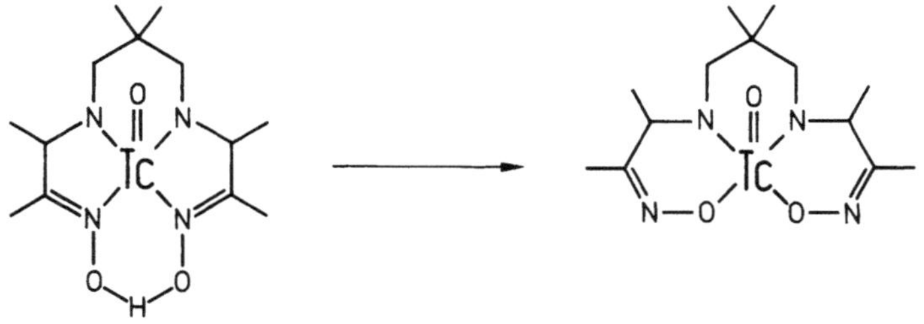

Fig. 8 Possible Tc-HM-PAO Re-arrangement reaction.

In an isotonic saline solution containing milligram quantities of free ligand the lipophilic complexes of this kind convert slowly to a hydrophilic species. In-vivo this conversion is accelerated by proteins and – after passage of the lipophilic compound through the BBB – the hydrophilic product is trapped inside the brain tissue. A large number of PAO-derivatives of this kind were synthesized and the physicochemical properties of their ^{99m}Tc-complexes and their in-vivo distribution studied. The selected ligand, HM-PAO combines good in-vitro stability with high brain-uptake and long-lasting retention in the brain. The retention of this class of converting compound in the brain of animals and humans has been amply demonstrated. Preliminary data on the extraction efficiency with which the compounds cross the BBB as well as comparisons with x-ray tomographic data and brain perfusion data obtained with ^{123}I-amphetamine indicate that this class of compounds represents the first ^{99m}Tc-labelled radiopharmaceuticals that will be useful for the routine investigation of regional cerebral blood flow in patients with suspected perfusion abnormalities, such as Alzheimer's and multi-infarct-dementias, tumour and stroke patients as well as for the evaluation of the cerebral vasculature patency in patients that are about to undergo carotid artery and cardiovascular surgical intervention.

References

[1] Volkert, W. A., D. E. Troutner, T. J. Hoffman et al.: ^{99m}Tc-propylene amine oxime; a potential brain radiopharmaceutical. J. Nucl. Med. **24** (1983) 128.

[2] Burns, H. D., R. F. Dannals, L. G. Marzilli et al.: Preparation and partial characterization of aminoethanethiol complexes of carrier free ^{99m}Tc, J. Nucl. Med., **20** (1979) 641.

[3] Yokoyama, A., Y. Terauchi, K. Horiuchi et al.: ^{99m}Tc-kethoxal-bis (thio-semicarbazone), an uncharged complex with a tetravalent ^{99m}Tc state and its excretion into bile. J. Nucl. Med. **17** (1976) 816–819.

[4] Holman, B. L., R. G. Lee, T. C. Hill et al: A comparison of two cerebral perfusion tracers, N-isopropyl ^{123}I-p-iodoamphetamine and ^{123}I-HIPDM, in the human. J. Nucl. Med. **25** (1984) 25–30.

[5] Von Schulthess, G. K., E. Ketz, P. A. Schubiger et al.: Regional quantitative noninvasive assessment of cerebral perfusion and function with N-isopropyl-[^{123}I]p-iodoamphetamine. J. Nucl. Med. **26** (1985) 9–16.

[6] Kung, H. F., M. Blau: Regional Intracellular pH shift: A proposed new mechanism for radiopharmaceutical uptake in brain and other tissues. J. Nucl. Med. **21** (1980) 147–152.

[7] Van Royen, E. A., J. F. De Bruine, A. Vyth et al.: ^{201}Tl-diethyldithio-carbamate (^{201}Tl-DDC): An alternative to ^{123}I-N-isopropyl-p-iodoamphetamine (^{123}I-IMP)? European nuclear Medicine Congress. Helsinki August 1984. Abstract 150, p. 144.

[8] Hansch, C., A. Leo: Substituent contants for correlation analysis in chemistry and biology. Wiley, New York 1979.

[9] Levin, Va. A.: Relationship of octanol/water partition Coefficient and molecular weight to rat brain capillary permeability. J. Med. Chem. **23** (1980) 682–684.

[10] Dischino, D. D., M. J. Welch, M.- R. Kilbourn et al.: Relationship between Lipophilicity and Brain extraction of ^{11}C-labelled Radiopharmaceuticals. J. Nucl. Med. **24** (1983) 1030–1038.

[11] Hansch, C., A. R. Steward, S. M. Anderson et al.: The parabolic dependence of drug action upon lipophilic character as revealed by a study of hypnotics. J. Med. Chem. **11** (1968) 1–11.

Potential New Approaches for the Development of Brain Imaging Agents for Single-Photon Applications

F. F. Knapp Jr., P. C. Srivastava

Introduction

^{123}I-labeled lipophilic radiopharmaceuticals which cross the intact blood-brain barrier and mimic regional blood flow [34] can potentially be used for scanning brain lesions by either planar or single photon computerized tomographic (SPECT) techniques [6]. After intravenous administration the delivery of such lipophilic substances to the brain is flow limited and the initial levels of cerebral radioactivity are thus proportional to regional perfusion. After equilibrium is reached, many agents are cleared or "washed out" from the brain tissue at a rate directly proportional to regional blood flow and many others show reversible permeability to the blood-brain barrier (freely enter and exit). Such agents are not optimal for brain imaging due to their rapid clearance. A variety of strategies have, therefore, been pursued to design agents which, will show rapid first-pass extraction, followed by rapid blood clearance with resulting good brain: blood ratios and exhibit prolonged cerebral retention with minimal redistribution. In this manner imaging technologies which take long acquisition periods, such as SPECT, can be used to qualitatively and potentially quantitatively determine the regional distribution of the tracer, which reflects blood perfusion.

One strategy that has been pursued is the screening of a variety of structurally-modified radioiodinated amphetamines [48, 49] which show high cerebral extraction. These studies have resulted in the development of p-[^{123}I]iodo-N-isopropylamphetamine (IMP) [26, 33] which is being used for SPECT studies in humans, and exhibits high cerebral extraction and slow wash-out. The amphetamines apparently bind strongly to high-affinity non-specific sites. Another strategy involves the "pH shift" agents, using radiolabeled amines that are "trapped" in the brain by the slightly lower cerebral pH in comparison to plasma [29, 30, 32]. The extension of this concept has resulted in the development of N,N,N'-trimethyl-N'-[2-hydroxy-3-methyl-[^{123}I]-iodobenzyl]-1,3-propanediamine (HIPDM) which also shows excellent properties in human studies [35].

^{123}I has excellent radionuclidic and chemical properties for use in diagnostic radiopharmaceuticals. The emission of the abundant (84%) 159 keV gamma photon allows the use of routinely available Anger-type cameras which are available in all nuclear medicine clinics. It is interesting to note that although the importance of ^{123}I has been discussed for two decades, only recently has the potential usefulness of this radionuclide really been demonstrated. The current interest and further development of tissue-specific ^{123}I-labeled radiopharmaceuticals have been catalyzed to a great extent by the successful use of [^{123}I]IMP. The dramatic increase in the number of papers presented at the American Society of Nuclear Medicine Meetings (fig. 1) can be attributed to recent developments with IMP and related agents and the

Fig. 1

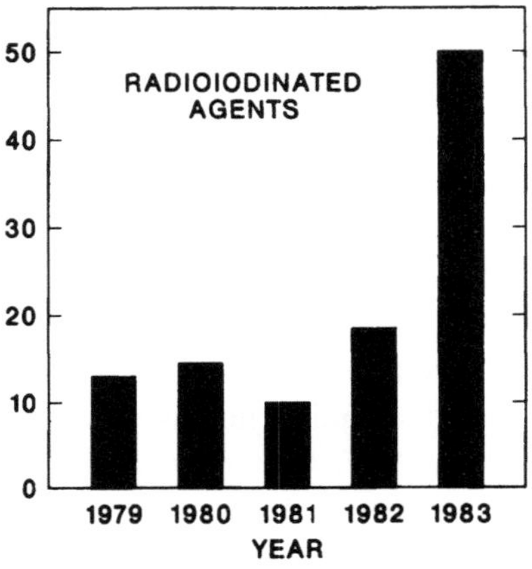

Fig. 2

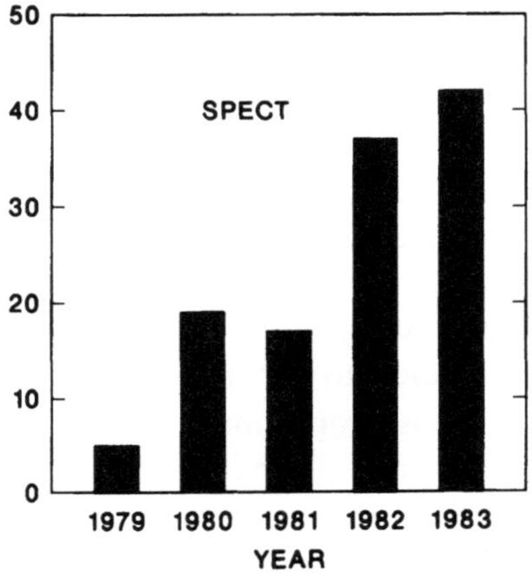

Fig. 1 Number of papers discussing radioiodinated agents at the U.S. Society of Nuclear Medicine Meetings from 1979–1983.

Fig. 2 Number of papers on single-photon computerized tomography (SPECT) presented at the U.S. Society of Nuclear Medicine Meetings from 1979 through 1983.

evaluation of chemical strategies for incorporation of this radionuclide into different tissue-specific agents. An additional index of the growth in this area is the increase in papers presented at these meetings using SPECT (fig. 2). It would appear that we are now on a threshold for the rapid increase in the development and use of ^{123}I-labeled agents. Not only are agents like [^{123}I]-IMP and ^{123}I-labeled fatty acids being more widely used, but the commercial availability of ^{123}I in the United States and Europe is rapidly increasing.

The goals of this paper are to describe new strategies being pursued at several institutions for the brain-specific delivery of radionuclides that can be used to evaluate regional cerebral perfusion by single photon imaging techniques. A comprehensive review of the literature is beyond the scope of these proceedings and our goal is to, therefore, present a description of several examples of interesting new strategies that have recently been reported. In addition, we also describe a new approach being pursued at our institution for the brain-specific delivery of radioiodinated iodophenylalkyl-substituted dihydronicotiamide systems which show good brain uptake and retention in preliminary studies in rats. Following transport into the brain these agents appear to undergo facile intracerebral oxidation to the quaternized analogues which do not cross the intact blood-brain-barrier and are effectively trapped in the brain.

New Methyl-Substituted Amphetamine Analogues

Investigators continue their search for molecules that can be modified and readily radiolabeled and evaluated as potential cerebral imaging agents. As described earlier, the excellent properties of ^{123}I give this radionuclide great promise for incorporation into brain-specific agents that can be used like IMP or HIPDM. In addition, the wide variety of radiolabeling methods which are useful for the incorporation of ^{123}I into these molecules further stimulates this area of research. From a structrual perspective, the iodine atom is about the size of a methyl group and can thus be introduced into tissue-specific molecules in many cases without drastically altering the size and shape or polarity of the molecule. This is in direct contrast to the presence of bulky chelating groups required to bind radionuclides which have more complex oxidation states, such as ^{99m}Tc. An example of important differences in chemical strategies and difficulties in incorporating the highly desirable ^{99m}Tc radionuclide into these types of agents is illustrated by the tremendous effort, as of yet unsuccessful, in preparing a ^{99m}Tc analogue of HIPDM [27, 28, 31]. Although the success of these efforts is highly desirable and will undoubtedly be achieved, the pursuit of ^{123}I-labeled agents continues.

The interesting properties and success with [^{123}I]IMP in clinical studies have prompted the evaluation of other structural analogues having the basic amphetamine structure in an effort to optimize structural features that may lead to higher cerebral retention and less redistribution and wash-out. An evaluation of the effects of α-dimethyl-branching on the cerebral extraction and retention properties of a structurally modified amphetamine analogue, phentermine (fig. 3), has recently been reported [8]. Phentermine (α,α-dimethylphenethylamine) is a potent sympathomimetric drug which is used as an anorexic [39]. The CNS effects of this agent suggested that p-iodinated analogues may retain these neurological properties and also show high cerebral uptake. In addition, the presence of geminal dimethyl-branching at the α-position would inhibit subsequent metabolism by interfering with transformation via the monoamine oxidase system (MAO) and other catabolic events. The p-[^{125}I]iodophentermine exhibited the expected high cerebral extraction

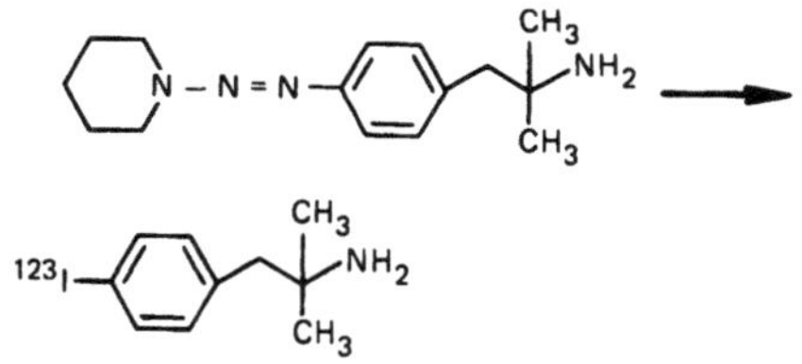

Fig. 3 Iodophentermine.

and retention in rats (1.7% dose/gm at 5 and 30 min) further confirmed by gamma camera imaging with the [^{123}I]-labeled analogue in dogs. This agent therefore shows good promise for further evaluation and a careful comparison with IMP and HIPDM to study the relative cerebral and lung uptake and retention properties should be pursued.

New Radioiodinated Nitrogen Heterocycles

An interesting class of radioiodinated nitrogen-containing heterocyclic agents which have recently been studied [18] are the N,N-disubstituted piperazines (fig. 4). The parent compound, piperazine, was used as early as the beginning of the twentieth century for the treatment of gout since it readily dissolved uric acid. A variety of aryl-substituted piperazines act on the central nervous system including "anti-aggressive" effects [16], "anti-hypertensive" activity [11, 17], and "neuroleptic" activity [21, 22]. The effects in the latter class are most pertinent to the current discussion of the potential use of radioiodinated arylpiperazines, since "Fluanison" is a methoxyphenylpiperazine-substituted butyrophenone that shows potent CNS activity. Another example is "Prazosin" (1-(4-amino-6,7-dimethoxy-2-quinazolinyl)-4-(2-furanylcarbonyl)-piperazine) an agent that also shows "antihypertensive" activity [7].

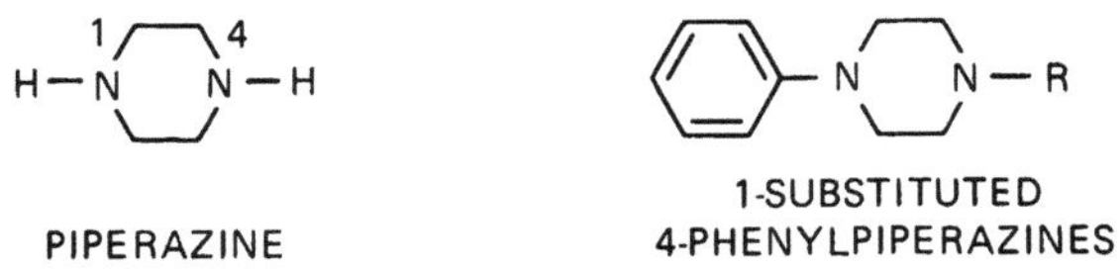

Fig. 4

The presence of two nitrogen atoms in the piperazine ring system allowed the preparation of a wide variety of nonsymmetrical N,N'-disubstituted piperazine derivatives. The N-aryl piperazine moiety represents a convenient group for the introduction and stabilization of radioiodide. Several N-(p-iodophenyl)-N'-substituted piperazine derivatives were prepared and the [^{125}I]-labeled analogues evaluated in rats (fig. 5). These interesting agents show good brain uptake and very high brain: blood ratios, although the relative distribution and retention properties of these analogues in other organs were not reported [18]. From the data reported, however, it would appear that a combination of optimal brain uptake and high brain: blood ratios are exhibited by the N'-alkyl-substituted analogue. The alicyclic analogue shows considerably less absolute brain uptake and the presence of more complex heterocyclic-carbonyl substituted N'-substituent does not seem to interfere with high cerebral extraction. Distribution data have only been reported, however, for 4 min after injection and these studies will undoubtedly be extended over a longer period of time to evaluate the important parameters of retention.

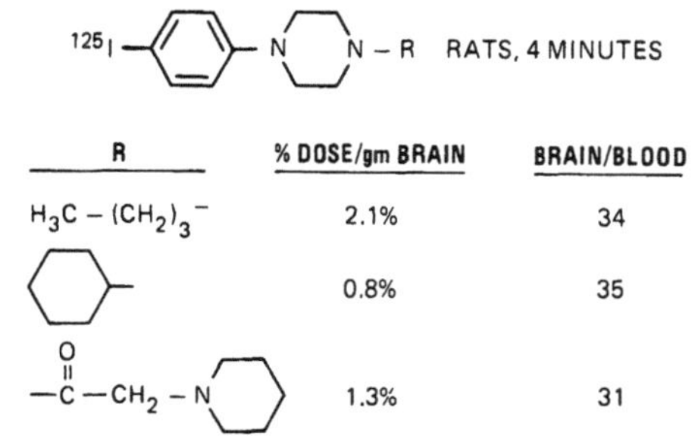

Fig. 5 Piperazine derivatives (% Dose/gm brain)

Thiocarbamic Acid Complexes of Cationic Radionuclides

There is also interest in important applications of complexes formed with cationic radionuclides since many metallic elements that have useful radionuclides can form complexes with organic agents that can determine the tissue distribution properties and thus target these agents for specific clinical applications. Complexes of both single photon and positron-emitting radionuclides can be prepared. Although the present discussion is focussed on single-photon radionuclides, it should be noted that efforts at several institutions are directed at developing lipid-soluble complexes with positron emitters such as ^{68}Ga [15, 25] and cryptate type compleces of ^{82}Rb [25]. These agents hold promise to evaluate both regional cerebral blood flow and myocardial perfusion. The development of these types of agents using positron-emitting radionuclides obtained from generator systems (^{82}Sr/^{82}Rb, ^{68}Ge/^{68}Ga, etc.) is very important since their availability would allow use with positron-emission tomographic devices at institutions that do not have a cyclotron.

Complexes with the single photon emitters would presumably have wider availability. An interesting and important observation has recently been reported involving the pronounced brain uptake of ^{201}Tl complexed with diethyldithiocarbamic acid (DDC). ^{201}Tl is the only widely available agent for the routine evaluation of regional coronary perfusion and for the differentiation of ischemia from infarction by comparison of stress and redistribution at rest. The whole body distribution of ^{201}Tl in man is well established and although [^{201}Tl]-chloride shows high myocardial, lung, kidney and thyroid uptake, ^{201}Tl does not cross the intact blood-brain barrier under normal conditions. The [^{201}Tl]DDC complex (fig. 6) is easily formed by reaction of [^{201}Tl]chloride with sodium diethyldithiocarbamate and forms a highly lipid-soluble complex that is easily extracted by organic solvents and can be analyzed by routine chromatographic methods. The mondentate [^{201}Tl]DDC complex also is highly soluble in physiological saline and can be administered immediately following preparation. This agent readily crosses the intact blood-brain barrier in rats [47] and rabbits [46] and shows high cerebral uptake and rapid blood clearance resulting in high brain: blood ratios. Although the use of DDC as a detoxification agent for thallicosis had been reported a number of years ago [44], this application has only recently been pursued. The possibility of cerebral concentration of [^{201}Tl]DDC was prompted by the reported increased neurological symptoms during NaDDC treatment of thallium intoxication [36]. Because of the ready availability of ^{201}Tl in nuclear medicine facilities, [^{201}Tl]DDC could represent a useful and widely available cerebral perfusion agent. A description of clinical studies with [^{201}Tl]DDC is included in another section of these proceedings [46].

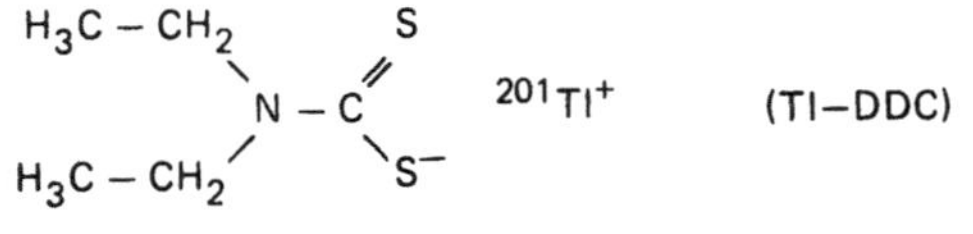

Fig. 6

The formation of high lipid-soluble complexes between metallic cations and DDC and related anions has been well known for a number of years [19, 37]. In fact, NaDDC extraction followed by further chemical separation and spectrophotometric analysis is a standard procedure for the analysis of trace elements in sea water [23, 24, 43]. The pH requirements, solubility and spectral properties of DDC complexes of many different metallic cations is well documented [19]. Since there are a variety of cationic metallic radionuclides that have attractive properties for diagnostic applications, it would appear at first glance that the use of DDC complexes of other radionuclides such as ^{111}In, ^{67}Ga, ^{64}Cu or ^{67}Cu, etc., would be possible. It appears, however, the ^{201}Tl is essentially a unique example of a highly aqueous soluble DDC complex since thallous ion is monovalent and thus forms a monodentate complex. We have prepared the tridentate [^{111}In]DDC_3 and [^{67}Ga]DDC_3, and bidentate [^{64}Cu]DDC_2 complexes, and as expected, they are very lipophilic and exhibit very low solubility in saline. Thus, unfortunately they cannot be used in the same elegant manner as [^{201}Tl]DDC to measure brain blood flow. However, there are a large number of structurally-modified thiolate ligands similar to DDC which may show higher aqueous solubility [37] and these should be explored to determine their potential usefulness in forming aqueous soluble complexes with other useful radionuclides.

We have recently evaluated the tissue distribution of [^{64}Cu]DDC in rats. As described earlier, copper (II) readily forms a highly lipid soluble Cu-DDC complex. ^{64}Cu is a very attractive isotope for potential use in diagnostic nuclear medicine since it is one of the few neutron-deficient radioisotopes which can be inexpensively produced in a nuclear reactor via neutron irradiation of the enriched ^{63}Cu by the ^{63}Cu(n,γ)^{64}Cu reaction. It is normally processed to give $^{64}CuCl_2$ [5]. While the monodentate Tl-DDC forms a complex which is lipophilic yet highly soluble in physiological saline, the high K_D value for $Cu(DDC)_2$ results in very low aqueous solubility. The [^{64}Cu]DDC was therefore complexed with 6% delipidated BSA and administered to rats (tab. 1). Although the plasma levels remained high, probably as a result from high affinity to ceruloplasmin, the [^{64}Cu]DDC complex showed considerably higher (4 to 6 fold) brain uptake than control studies with [^{64}Cu]-Cl_2. We have also prepared similar [^{111}In]$(DDC)_3$ and [^{67}Ga]$(DDC)_3$ complexes but these tridentate agents are difficult to formulate and show low brain uptake, presumably at least partly due to their very high lipid solubility. Nonetheless, the evaluation of structurally-modified dithiocarbamate complexes should be pursued since other neutral, yet more aqueous soluble agents, may show useful biodistribution properties and promise for radiopharmaceutical applications. As an example, the bis-ethanol dithiocarbamate complex of Cu (II) has been reported to show aqueous solubility [13, 38].

Table 1 Brain and blood levels of radioactivity after intravenous administration of $^{64}CuCl_2$ and [^{64}Cu] copperdiethyldithiocarbamate ([^{64}Cu]DDC_2) to female Fischer Rats

Agent, Time	Percent dose/gm Brain	 Blood
^{64}Cu-DDC		
5 min	0.40–0.60	1.93–2.21
60 min	0.28–0.31	0.86–0.94
$^{64}CuCl_2$		
5 min	0.10–0.11	1.62–2.26
60 min	0.05–0.05	0.73–0.82

Radioiodinated Iodophenyl-alkyl-Substituted Dihydronicotinamide Systems

A new approach for brain specific sustained release of therapeutic drugs has recently been described by Bodor et al. [1, 2, 3] which involves the chemical transformation (fig. 7) of the quaternary form of a drug [Q^+], which normally does not penetrate the blood-brain barrier, to a reduced lipid soluble form [HQ]. After intravenous administration the lipid soluble [HQ) is readily distributed throughout the body and easily crosses the intact blood-brain barrier. The NAD ⇄ NADH oxidation, however, regenerates the original impermeable form [Q^+] from [HQ] within the brain. This results in a unique "trapping" of the parent drug in the brain (intracellular pool). This approach has been successfully used for the cerebral delivery of dopamine to rats [1, 2]. We have further extended these studies to evaluate the potential utility of this unique approach for the cerebral delivery of radiopharmaceuticals as a means to potentially measure regional cerebral perfusion as described below [40, 45]. It was anticipated that the hydrophilic [Q^+] would be "trapped" in the brain and rapidly cleared from the blood and other body tissues. This would result in high brain uptake and acceptable brain: blood ratios required for optimal brain imaging. As a part of our interest in the development of new brain imaging agents, the goals of the present study were to develop a chemical approach to

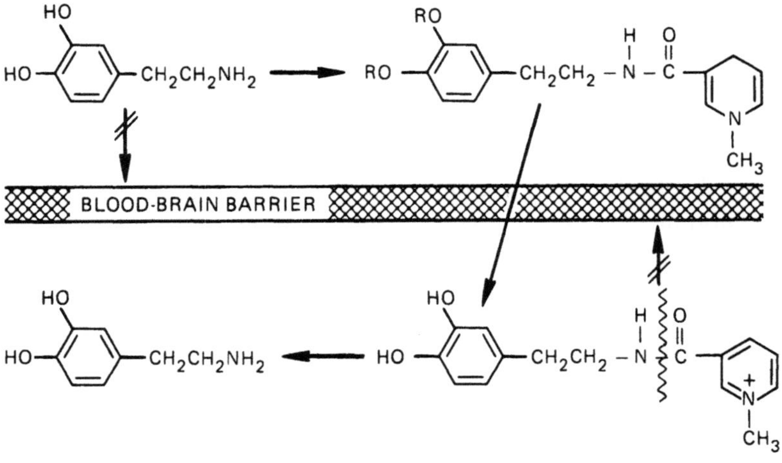

Fig. 7

prepare model [^{125}I]-labeled phenylalkylamines linked to a dihydropyridine carrier and to evaluate the biodistribution properties of these agents in rats.

A radioiodinated moiety such as p-iodophenethylamine coupled with dihydropyridine in the lipid soluble form (8a, Scheme I) should be transported across the blood-brain barrier and oxidized to the quaternary form (7a) within the brain and thus remain "trapped". At this stage the CO-NH bond could also be potentially cleaved by the NAD ⇄ NADH system to regenerate the radioiodinated phenylethylamine. For preliminary tissue distribution studies in rats the model radioiodinated compound, 1-methyl-3-[N-[β-(4-iodophenyl)ethyl]carbamoyl]-1,4-dihydropyridine(8a), was prepared as shown in Scheme I. Condensation of nicotinic acid (1) with N-hydroxysuccinimide (2) in dimethylformamide (DMF) in the presence of dicyclohexylcarbodimide (DCC) gave the activated ester, N-succinimidyl pyridine-3-carboxylate (3) as a useful intermediate for the formation of "CONH" bond when coupled with amines [41]. Quaternization of (3) with methyl iodide and coupling with p-aminophenyl-ethylamine gave 1-methyl-3-[N-[β-(p-aminophenyl)ethyl]carbamoyl] pyridinium iodide (5). Diazo coupling of (5) with piperidine or diethylamine at 0° C using hydrofluoric acid (HF, 48%) and sodium nitrite gave the alicyclic or diethyl triazene substrates (6) without an intramolecular cyclization with the carboxamide group [20]. Triazene decomposition with sodium iodide (Na[^{125}I]) and anhydrous HF in acetone at 0° C readily furnished 1-methyl-3[N-[β-(4-[^{125}I]iodophenyl)ethyl]carbamoyl]pyridinium iodide [^{125}I] (7a), the [Q^+] form of the product. Sodium dithionite reduction of [^{125}I] (7a) then provided the desired compound [^{125}I] (8a). In order to evaluate the relative in vivo susceptibility to oxidation and subsequent brain uptake of model dihydropyridine carriers, an 4-[^{125}I]iodoaniline coupled model agent, 1-methyl-3-N-(4-[^{125}I]iodophenyl)carbamoyl-1,4-dihydropyridine [^{125}I] (8b), was also prepared as shown in Scheme I. Nucleophilic attack by the amino group of p-iodoaniline on the activated ester (4) gave 1-methyl-N-3-(p-iodophenyl)-carbamoylpyridinium iodide (7b). Because of synthetic considerations, in this case, the p-radioiodide was fabricated prior to coupling the amine with the activated ester (4). ^{125}I-labeled p-iodoaniline was prepared by $[^{125}I]I_2$ treatment of commercially available 4-aminophenylmercuric acetate following a general method developed in our laboratory for the synthesis of radioiodinated compounds from the corresponding mercuric acetate precursors [42].

The tissue distribution of radioiodinated compounds $[^{125}I]$ (7a) and $[^{125}I]$ (8a) was evaluated in rats. The quaternary compound (7a) showed very low brain uptake whereas the lipophilic, dihydro compound (8a) exhibited significantly higher brain

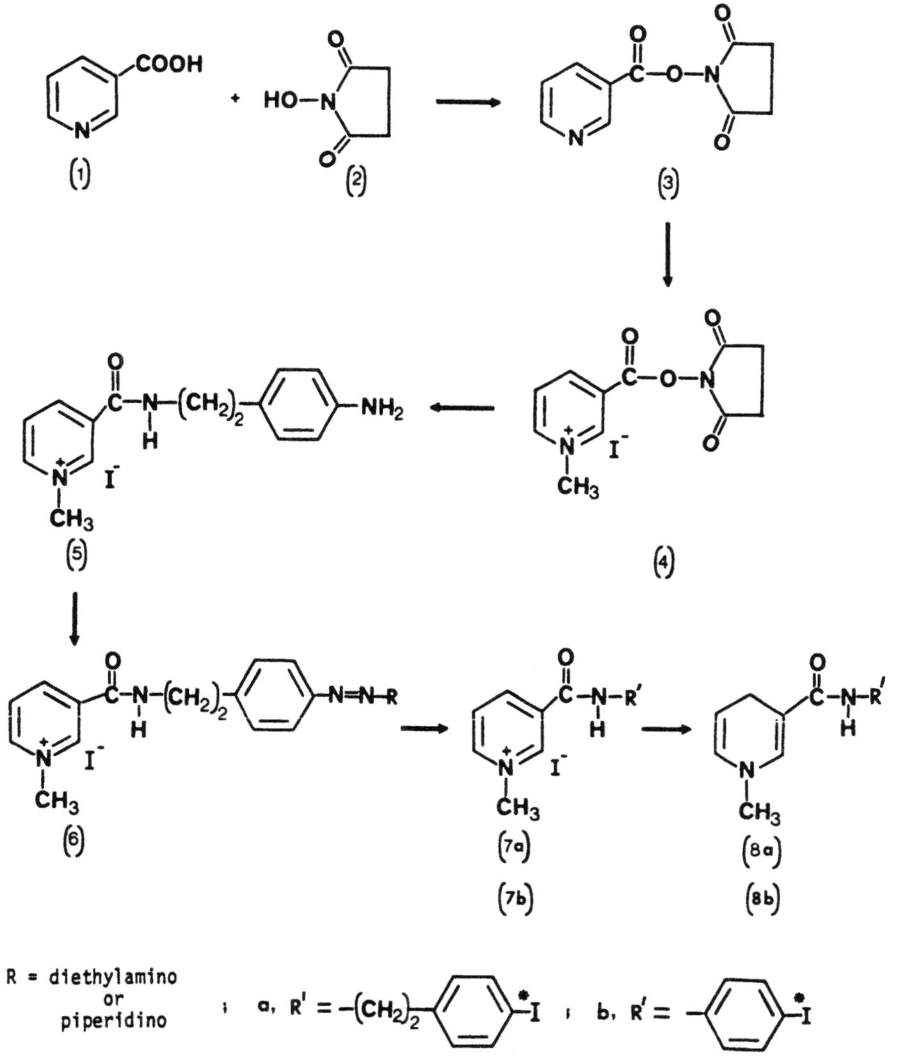

Scheme 1

uptake, as expected from the studies reported by Bodor et al. [1, 2, 3]. Our studies with model radioiodinated agents further confirm that structurally-modified, reduced compounds (e. g. 8) more easily cross the blood-brain barrier as compared to the parent, quaternary drugs e. g. (7).

Oxidation of the oxygen sensitive dihydro products (8a) and (8b) was inhibited, prior to injection, by addition of vitamin E as a stabilizer. Vitamin E was also added to [^{125}I] (7) prior to administration as a control and to evaluate any effect of vitamin E on the tissue distribution of [^{125}I] (8). As expected, the quaternary compound (7a) showed low brain uptake and high activity in the blood pool (fig. 8), whereas the

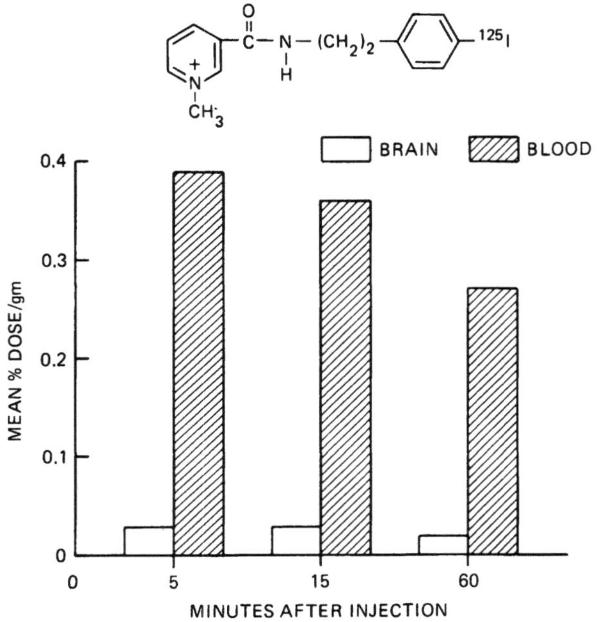

Fig. 8 Comparison of the relative brain and blood levels (mean % dose/gm) after administration of [^{125}I] (7a) to Sprague-Dawley rats.

lypophilic, dihydro compound (8a) showed significant brain uptake (fig. 9), and exhibited good brain: blood ratios. ^{125}I-labeled 4-iodoaniline, itself, has been reported to exhibit brain uptake (0.47%/gm, 5 min) and rapid clearance (0.03%/gm, 60 min) in rats. In our studies, 4-[^{125}I]iodoaniline showed similar distribution properties (uptake and clearance) in rats. Superior distribution properties of [^{125}I] (8b) as compared to 4-[^{125}I]iodoaniline clearly demonstrate that coupling of such radioiodinated amines with dihydropyridine carrier may be an effective way to achieve high uptake and retention in the brain.

These preliminary studies have demonstrated that dihydropyridine-linked lipophilic agents [^{125}I] (8a) and [^{125}I] (8b) cross the blood brain barrier and are quaternized within the brain preventing their release. The quaternary forms [^{125}I] (7a) and [^{125}I]

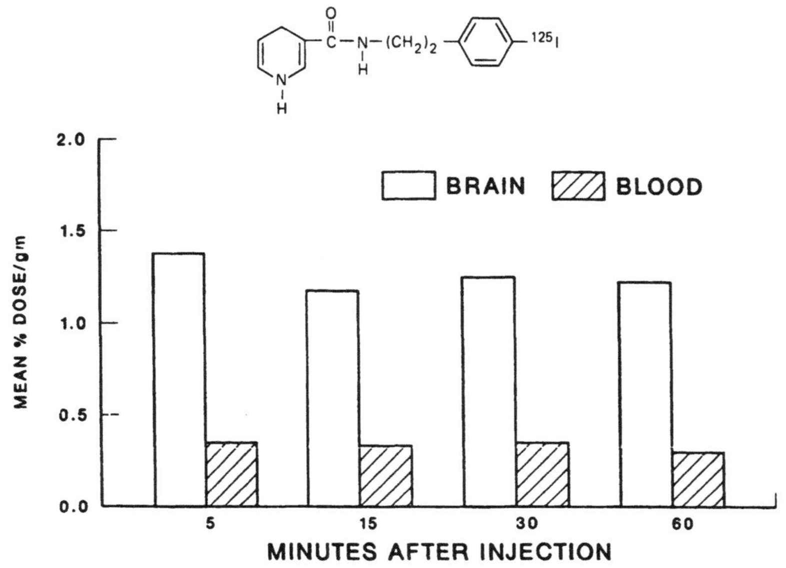

Fig. 9 Comparison of the relative brain and blood levels (mean % dose/gm) after administration of [^{125}I] (8a) to Sprague-Dawley rats.

(7b), however, cannot cross the blood-brain barrier and thus show low brain uptake. We have also shown that the facile oxidation of dihydropyridine compounds to the corresponding quaternary compounds on storage or prior to *in vivo* administration can be inhibited by adding vitamine E as a stabilizer. These studies have shown that brain-specific delivery of radiopharmaceuticals using the Boder approach is possible. In addition, these data also suggest that a more detailed evaluation of the brain specific sustained release of radiopharmaceuticals for potential application in evaluation of regional cerebral blood perfusion should be pursued.

Summary

A variety of new strategies for the development of cerebral perfusion agents radiolabeled with single-photon emitters are being pursued. There is still considerable interest in the use of ^{123}I and the commercial availability of this radionuclide is increasing. In addition to the ^{123}I-labeled agents, the recent success with the interesting [^{201}Tl]DDC complex may well be a prelude to the development and evaluation of other useful neutral and tissue specific complexes of cationic radionuclides. It is important for radiopharmacuetical scientists and clinical investigators to continue to closely interact and work together to effectively communicate the specific requirements of agents for applications for the measurement of regional cerebral perfusion.

Acknowledgements

This research was sponsored by the Office of Health and Environmental Research, U.S. Department of Energy under contract DE-AC05-840R21400 with Martin Marietta Energy Systems, Inc. The authors thank H. Biersack, M. D., his colleagues and the Rheinisch-Westfälische Gesellschaft für Nuclearmedizin for the opportunity to participate in this symposium held in Bonn on October 12–13, 1984. The authors thank L. S. Ailey for typing the manuscript.

References

[1] Bodor, N., H. H. Farag: J. Med. Chem. **26** (1983a) 313.
[2] Bodor, N., H. H. Farag: J. Med. Chem. **26** (1983b) 528.
[3] Bodor, N., J. W. Simpkins: Science **221** (1983) 65.
[4] Brooks, R. R., B. J. Presley, I. R. Kaplan: Talanta **14** (1967) 809.
[5] Brown, L. C., A. P. Callahan: Int. J. Appl. Radiat. Isot. **23** (1972) 535.
[6] Budinger, T. F.: J. Nucl. Med. **21** (1980) 279.
[7] Cohen, J.: J. Clin. Pharmacol. J. New Drugs **10** (1970) 408.
[8] Elmaleh, D. R., H. Kizuka, G. Boudreaux et al.: Proceedings of the 5th International Radiopharmaceutical Chemistry Symposium, Tokyo, Japan, July 1984. J. Lab. Cmpds. and RAdiopharm. XXI, p. 88, 1078 (1984).
[9] Fazio, F., P. Gerundini, G. C. Lenzi: J. Nucl. Med. **24** (1983) 5 (abst).
[10] Forne, F. E., A. R. Foquet, M. A. Scarispan et al.: ES (Spanish Patent) 502, 469 (CA 98, 16, 727B, 1983).
[11] Fregnan, B., R. Porta: Arzneimittel-Forsch. 31 (1981) 70, for biochemical and behavioral effects.
[12] Fukushi, K., T. Irie, O. Inoue et al.: Proceedings of the 5th International Radiopharmaceutical Chemistry Symposium Tokyo, Japan, July 1984, J. Lab. Cmpds and Radiopharm. XXI, p. 90 (1984).
[13] Geiger, E., H. G. Muller: Helv. Chim. Acta **26** (1943) 996.
[14] Goodman, L. S., A. Gilman (eds.): The Pharmacological Basis of Therapeutics, 4th ed., The MacMillian Co., New York 1970.
[15] Green, M. A., C. J. Mathias, M. Welch: Proceedings of the 5th International Radiopharmaceutical Chemistry Symposium Tokyo, Japan, July 1984, J. Lab. Cmpds and Radiopharm. XXI, p. 9 (1984).
[16] Haeck, H. H., F. C. Hiller: Eur. Patent 48, 045 (Chem. Abst. **97** 38, 596G, 1982).
[17] Hampton, B. L., C. B. Pollard: J. Am. Chem. Soc. **54** (1937) 2570.
[18] Hanson, R. N., T. El-Shounbagy, M. Hasson: Proceedings of the 5th International Radiopharmaceutical Chemistry Symposium Tokyo, Japan, July 1984. J. Lab. Cmpds and Radiopharm. XXI, p. 92 (1984).
[19] Hulanicki, A.: Talanta **14** (1967) 1371.
[20] Ivanovics, G. A., R. J. Rousseau, M. Kawana et al.: J. Org. Chem. **39** (1974) 3651.
[21] Janssen, P. A. J., U. S. Patant, 2, 997, 472 (1961).
[22] Janssen, P. A. J., C. J. E. Niemegeers, K. H. L. Schellehens: Arznein. Forschungs. **15** (1965) 104.
[23] Kinrade, J. D., J. C. Van Loon: Anal. Chem. **46** (1974) 1894.
[24] Kremling, K., H. Petersen: Anal. Chim. Acta **70** (1974) 35.
[25] Krohn, K. A., Y. Yano, T. F. Budinger et al.: In: Radionuclide Generators – New Systems for Nuclear Medicine Applications (F. F. Knapp, Jr., T. A. Butler, eds.). American Chemical Society Symposium Series 241, Washington, D.C. (1984).
[26] Kuhl, D. E., J. R. Barrio, S. C. Huang et al.: J. Nucl. Med. **23** (1982) 196.

[27] Kung, H., M. Molnar, J. Billings et al.: J. Nucl. Med. **25** (1984a) 326.
[28] Kung, H. F., C. C. Yu, J. Billings et al.: Proceedings of the 5th International Radiopharmaceutical Chemistry Symposium Tokyo, Japan, July 1984, J. Lab. Cmpds. and Radiopharm. XXI, 24 (1984b).
[29] Kung, H. F., M. Blau: J. Nucl. Med. **21** (1980a) 147.
[30] Kung, H. F., M. Blau: J. Med. Chem. **23** (1980b) 1127.
[31] Kung, H. F., K. M. Tramposch, M. Blau: J. Nucl. Med. **24** (1983) 66.
[32] Lasser, N. A., L. Hendriksen, S. Holm: J. Nucl. Med. **24** (1983) 17.
[33] Lee, G. E., T. C. Hill, B. L. Holman et al.: Radiology **145** (1982) 795.
[34] Oldendorf, W. H.: Proc. Soc. Exp. Biol. Med. **19** (1974) 1182.
[35] Polak, J. F., B. L. Holman, J.-L. Moretti et al.: J. Nucl. Med. **25** (1984) 495.
[36] Rauws, A. G., M. Ten Ham, H. M. Kamerbeek: Arch. Int. Pharmacodyn. **182** (1969) 425.
[37] Sandell, E. B., H. Onishi (eds.): Photometric Determination of Trace Metals, General Aspects. Fourth Edition, John Wiley and Sons, Chapter 6F, pp. 504–579, 1979 (review).
[38] Serfass, H. J., W. S. Levine: Chem. Anal. **36** (1967) 55.
[39] Shelton, R. S., M. G. Van Campen: U.S. Patent 2, 408, 345 (1946).
[40] Srivastava, P. C., M. L. Tedjamulia, F. F. Knapp, jr.: 188th Amer. Chem. Sos. National Meeting, Philadelphia, Pennsylvania, August 26–31, 1984 (abstract).
[41] Srivastava, P. C., R. W. Mancuso, R. J. Rousseau et al.: J. Med. Chem. **71** (1974) 1207.
[42] Srivastava, P. C., F. F. Knapp, Jr., G. W. Kabalka et al.: Synth. Comm. (in press, 1985).
[43] Sturgeon, R. E., S. S. Berman, A. Desaulniers et al.: Talanta **27** (1980) 85.
[44] Sunderman, F. W.: Am. J. Med. Sci., **253** (1967) 209.
[45] Tedjamulia, M. L., P. C. Srivastava, F. F. Knapp, Jr.: J. Med. Chem. (submitted 1985).
[46] Van Royen, E. A., J. F. de Bruine, A. Vyth et al.: In: Nuclear Medicine in Research and Practice, European nuclear Medicine Congress, Helsinki, Finland, August 1984, p. 144–145 (abstract).
[47] Vyth, A., P. J. Fennema, J. B. van der Schoot: Pharm. Weekblad Sci. Ed. **5** (1983) 213.
[48] Winchell, H. S., R. M. Baldwin, T. H. Lin: J. Nucl. Med. **21** (1982) 940.
[49] Winchell, H. S., W. D. Horst, L. Braun et al.: J. Nucl. Med. **21** (1980) 947.

Performance of a Multidetector Brain Scanner Compared to a Rotating Gamma Camera System for the Same Scan Task

S. P. Mueller, S. C. Moore, B. L. Holman

Interest in nuclear medicine brain scanning has been revived with the introduction of new gamma-emitting tracers such as ^{123}I N-isopropyl-iodo-amphetamine (IMP) or ^{123}I 3-Quinuclidinyl 4-iodobenzilate (QNB) for assessing the distribution of blood flow or receptor binding sites in the brain using single photon emission computed tomography (SPECT).

The tracer uptake corresponding to physiologic function in the brain yields a high contrast distribution in different brain structures. Both the scientific investigation of these new agents and their application in clinical routine require, first, the identification of these brain structures, which are generally small compared to the resolution of current SPECT systems; and, second, assessment of size, shape and regional uptake, ideally in a quantitative manner. It is known that these "higher order" imaging tasks require a high resolution in order to optimize observer performance in the presence of statistical noise [1]. Therefore, high-resolution, low-noise SPECT systems are required. This has prompted comparisons of existing SPECT scanners in terms of extrapolated sensitivity for a resolution and slice thickness of 1 cm [2]. However, the image noise is not uniquely determined by the count sensitivity of a system: this is because count sensitivity does not describe the effects of the reconstruction filter on noise and resolution.

Recent work has demonstrated the inadequacy of describing the image noise for a special-purpose multidetector brain scanner simply in terms of the count sensitivity [6]. A comparative re-evaluation of this system is therefore necessary.

We will compare the resolution and noise for the required 3-dimensional (3D) reconstruction for the multidetector scanner with a current state-of-the-art rotating gamma camera system.* Two collimators have been studied with the gamma camera; a low-energy, all-purpose (LEAP) collimator and a medium-energy, high-resolution long bore (LB) collimator (tab. 1).

The multi-detector brain scanner contains 12 rectangular detectors with short focal-length (25 cm) point-focusing collimators. Each detector scans through half the

* General Electric 400 AT.

Table 1 Dimensions of the collimators for the rotating gamma camera

	LEAP	LB
collimator thickness	41 mm	130 mm
hole shape	hexagonal	hexagonal
hole diameter (face to face)	2.5 mm	4.4 mm
septa thickness	0.3 mm	0.18 mm
manufacturing method	cast	foil
field of view	41 cm diameter	26×39 cm

field-of-view. The focal point moves tangentially along 6 parallel lines; the innermost is in the center of the field of view. At the end of a scan line each detector is incremented by 2.1 cm radially to scan the next tangential line. Two opposing detectors, therefore, acquire a set of 11 parallel lines through the entire field of view. (The midline is scanned by both detectors.) The 12 detectors simultaneously acquire six angular projections. Then the detector assembly is rotated twice by 10 degrees; at each angle six more angular projctions are collected [5]. Therefore, a complete set of projection data for one slice consists of 18 angular views of 11 scan lines each.

Each detector's crystal measures 20 × 12.5 × 2.5 cm. The longest side is parallel to the patient axis. Hence, the direction of greatest focusing of the collimator is across the image plane. Fig. 1 illustrates the relationship between the envelope of the collimator response function, i.e., the space that is "seen" by the detector, and the plane to be imaged. It is evident that only a small fraction of the detected counts emanates from the image plane itself when an axially extended object (such as the brain) is scanned with this system.

The 2-D reconstruction algorithm originally provided by the manufacturer filtered the data with a one-dimensional, rolled-off ramp filter along the tangential scan lines. The filtered projections were rotated and added into the reconstruction matrix using bi-linear interpolation. This algorithm did not take any out-of-slice effects into account.

It has recently been shown that the original reconstruction was only correct for sources with infinite cylindrical symmetry (where every slice looks the same). If more realistic source distributions are scanned, artifacts will be introduced. For example, the reconstruction of a homogeneous 1.5 cm thick disk with 15 cm diameter has more than a 20% bowl shaped "dip" in the center [6].

In order to obtain an accurate reconstruction of a slice through an object of arbitrary shape, scans must be taken at multiple axial positions and each slice of interest corrected for the out-of-slice counts obtained. An analytical inversion of the unattenuated Radon transform for this scan geometry has been obtained [6].

The resulting 3-D reconstruction algorithm performs a 3-D Fourier transform (over the tangential, radial and axial directions) of each projection's data. These trans-

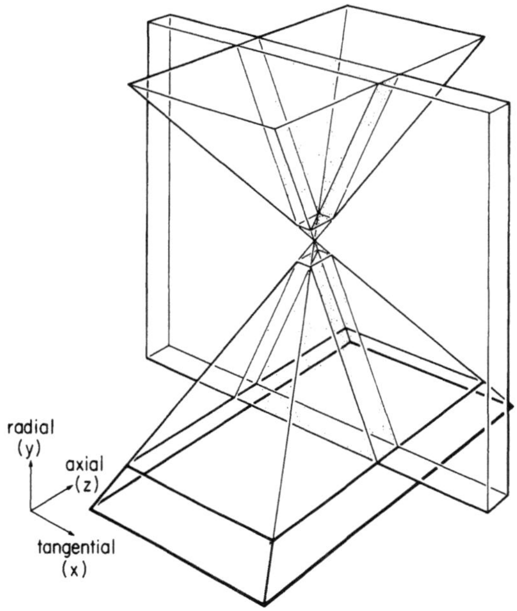

Fig. 1 The collimated detector, shown at the bottom, receives counts from the region inside the double-pyramid formed by the outer envelope of the collimator response. The contribution from the slice-of-interest is shaded. Most of the counts from an axially extended object emanate from out-of-slice locations. The analytical 3-D-recontruction puts these counts back where they belong in a volume of interest. In theory, the algorithm needs projection data from all axial and radial scan positions where the object-of-interest can be "seen" by the detector. Therefore, for an ideal reconstruction, the scan range in the axial and radial directions should increase with larger diameter and axial extent of the object.

formed projections are filtered with a 3-D filter and inverse transformed. The filtered 3-D angular projections are then rotated and put back into the reconstruction matrix. It was shown by Moore et al. [6] that the filter functions are mathematically well-behaved and reduce to the simpler 2-D reconstruction for the case of an object with infinite cylindrical symmetry. These operations are analogous to the filtered-backprojection algorithm for parallel beam geometry, where the measured projection data are filtered and backprojected to obtain an estimate of the original object.

The 3-D reconstruction provided an accurate image of the thin disk, if a least 5 slices on both sides of each slice-of-interest are used by the reconstruction. In order to reconstruct an infinite cylinder, however, additional tangential scan lines furthers away from the object had to be measured to satisfy mathematical requirements of the 3-D reconstruction.

To obtain the same %RMS noise in both the thin disk (reconstructed with the 3-D method) and the long cylinder (reconstructed with the 2-D method), it was necessary to scan the disk source 10 times longer than the cylinder. This lower effective sensitivity resulted from the requirement of scanning 11 slices of the disk just to reconstruct one central slice, as well as the different noise amplification of the 3-D method. Since the single-slice *count* sensitivity, measured with a long 15 cm diameter cylinder, was previously reported to be 12 000 cps μCi^{-1} ml [10], we conclude that the true noise-equivalent, single-slice sensitivity of this scanner (with the necessary 3-D method) is 1200 cps μCi^{-1} ml.

For the clinical situation of brain scanning, however, the single-slice noise-equivalent sensitivity is not meaningful. As the required number of slices-of-interest increases, the fraction of the total scan time spent scanning the additional 10 slices outside the volume of interest decreases.

This is fundamentally different than a parallel-collimated, rotating gamma camera, for which the noise in an individual slice is independent of the adjacent slices and the number of slices scanned.

In this paper we will compare the performance of the multi-detector scanner and the rotating gamma camera for scanning a 15 cm diameter, 7.5 cm long cylinder, representing the brain. Both systems will be compared for a total scan time of 43 minutes, corresponding to 64 angular samples and 40 sec/projection as currently used on the rotating camera.

Simulations

Resolution, slice thickness and %RMS noise for the 3-D-reconstruction on the multidetector brain scanner were determined from simulated data without including effects of attenuation and scatter. The collimator response function was generated by a Monte Carlo simulation to closely resemble the actual scanner. The tangential (x) resolution was 7.1 mm FWHM and the axial (z) resolution 15.2 mm FWHM for the simulated collimator, compared to 7 mm and 15 mm, respectively, measured on our scanner. In a subsequent Monte Carlo simulation this modelled collimator was used to scan a short axial line segment of 1.5 cm at multiple overlapping axial positions, spaced by 0.75 cm. We obtained raw data for 1.5 cm thick disk with 15 cm diameter by 2-D convolution of the short line source data with a circle of 15 cm diameter. Raw data for a 20 cm long, 15 cm diameter cylinder were correspondingly generated from a Monte Carlo simulation of a 20 cm long line source. The disk and the cylinder were normalized to have the same activity.

Noise-free line source data were reconstructed with the 3-D-reconstruction using the following combinations of Hanning window cutoffs for the tangential (k_x) und axial (k_z) spatial frequencies: (1) k_x cutoff = 1.333 cm^{-1}, no k_z window, (2) k_x cutoff = 0.6 cm^{-1}, no k_z window and (3) k_x cutoff = 0.6 cm^{-1}, k_z cutoff = 0.6 cm^{-1}. The maximum of a profile through the reconstructed point source image was estimated from a paraboloid through the highest three points and the FWHM calculated by linear interpolation. The slice thickness was determined from the maximum at different axial positions and deconvolved for the finite length of the short line source. These calculations were carried out for all three window combinations.

After adding Gaussian noise to the raw data, 3-D reconstructions of the simulated disk were performed with the same three windows described for the line source reconstruction and the %RMS noise was determined in a large square region in the center.

Phantom studies

Resolution and noise for both collimators on the rotating gamma camera were measured from phantom experiments and, therefore, include scatter and attenuation.

Resolution was determined from a 0.58 mm inner diameter line source filled with ^{99m}Tc, and suspended at the center of a 20 cm diameter water filled phantom. We acquired 128 projections in a 128 × 128 matrix and reconstructed the image using a filtered back-projection algorithm without attenuation correction. The FWHM was determined (as described for the simulations) both for images reconstructed using a Hanning window with a 0.8 cm^{-1} cutoff and without apodization, (i.e., ramp filter).

The LB collimator was operated at a radius-of-rotation of 17 cm, the LEAP at 22 cm. These distances allow the camera to clear the patients' shoulders in the clinical setting of brain SPECT.

The %RMS noise was measured in a 20 cm diameter cylindrical phantom filled with an activity concentration of 1 μCi/ml which approximates the average concentration of ^{123}I-iodoamphetamine in the brain. We acquired 64 projections in a 64 × 64 matrix format and reconstructed by filtered backprojection using Sorenson's attenuation correction. Data were acquired for 1, 2, 5, 10, 15, 30, 45, 60, and 90 seconds per projection. The %RMS noise in the reconstructed image was fitted to the equation: $\%RMS = c(N_{tot})^{-1/2}$. To reconstruct the images, we used the same two filters just described for the line source reconstruction, as well as a 3-D Hanning window with 0.8 cm^{-1} cutoff applied after tomographic reconstruction with an unwindowed ramp filter.

Results

Multidetector

Resolution and slice thickness, measured in images of the line segment reconstructed with the 3-D algorithm, are given in table 2. The FWHM resolution of 1.07 cm for a k_x-cutoff of 1.333 cm^{-1} is in good agreement with the resolution measured as 1.01 cm with a long line source using the original 2-D reconstruction algorithm for the real scanner [10].

Table 2 Performance parameters (measured and predicted) for SPECT systems compared. The rotating gamma camera data were measured using a 20 cm diameter cylindrical phantom and include the effects of scatter and attenuation. The results for the multi-detector scanner were obtained from attenuation-free simulations of a 1.5 cm thick, 15 cm diameter disk. The measured data were used to predict the %RMS noise from scanning a 7.5 cm long, 15 cm diameter cylinder (1μCi/ml) for a total scan time of 43 minutes (see text).

system	roll off window	cutoff frequency (cm^{-1})	in-slice resolution FWHM (cm)	slice thickness FWHM (cm)	noise amplification $c \times 10^3$	predicted %RMS noise 7.5 cm long 15 cm diameter phantom
Rotating gamma camera LEAP	–	no rolloff	1.96	2.0	11.0	7.7
(22 cm radius of rotation)	Hanning	0.8	2.30	2.0	3.8	2.6
	3-D-Hanning	0.8	2.30	2.3	2.5	1.8
Rotating gamma camera LB	–	no rolloff	1.27	1.3	10.4	12.8
(17 cm radius of rotation)	Hanning	0.8	1.75	1.3	3.6	4.5
	3-D-Hanning	0.8	1.75	1.8	2.8	3.4
Multidetector scanner	Hanning K_X / K_Z	1.333 / no rolloff	1.07	1.5	24.0	6.1
	Hanning K_X / K_Z	0.6 / no rolloff	1.83	1.5	6.7	1.7
(3-D-reconstruction)	Hanning K_X / K_Z	0.6 / 0.6	1.84	2.0	4.9	1.3

Images of the disk were reconstructed using 10.5×10^6 total counts obtained from 11 axial scan positions. The 3-D reconstruction with a k_x-cutoff of 1.333 cm^{-1} and no k_z-apodization produced an image noice of 7.4% RMS. Decreasing the k_x-cutoff to 0.6 cm^{-1} yielded 2.1% noise. Additional k_z windowing with a cutoff at 0.6 cm^{-1} increased the slice thickness from 1.5 cm to 2.0 cm and reduced the noise to 1.5%. Scanning a slice through a long cylinder containing the same activity concentration produced 5.0×10^6 total counts.

Rotating gamma camera

The measured resolution for both collimators is given in table 2. It is evident that the medium-energy, high-resolution LB collimator is superior to the LEAP. Its resolution when reconstructing with a 0.8 cm^{-1} Hanning window is better than the resolution of the LEAP when reconstructing without any rolloff. For a given axial window rolloff, the slice thickness given in table 2 is assumed to be the same as the in-slice resolution resulting from the same window applied during tomographic reconstruction. Thus, if no axial windowing is used, the slice thickness equals the in-slice resolution from a unwindowed reconstruction. For the 3-D Hanning window the slice thickness is the same as the in-slice resolution reconstructed with a 0.8 cm^{-1} cutoff.

The %RMS noise, described as a function of total counts in the image, is also shown in table 2. Note that the noise amplification constant, c, which describes the %RMS noise for the same total number of counts, is 3.6×10^3 for the LB collimator with a Hanning windowed ($k_x = 0.8\ cm^{-1}$) reconstruction while the LEAP yields 11.0×10^3 without apodization window.

Using the 20 cm diameter, ^{99m}Tc-filled phantom, the count sensitivity for the LB collimator was found to be 163 cps μCi^{-1} ml and 509 cps μCi^{-1} ml for the LEAP.

Discussion

Multidetector

The noise equivalent sensitivity for imaging arbitrarily shaped objects is difficult to extrapolate from our simulations of the thin disk. In the theory, [6] an integration from $-\infty$ to $+\infty$ has to be carried out over the entire function-space to allow the analytical inversion of the Radon-transform. This corresponds to scanning far away from the object in all 3-dimensions until the object is not "seen" anymore by the detectors, i.e., the detected counts are at the background level. If this requirement is not met, it means the data will be truncated and artifacts will be introduced. In general, this mathematical requirement of scanning areas where extremely low count rates are detected (to avoid truncation errors) is opposed to the goal of high sensitivity, which requires high count rates at all times during a scan.

Our simulation has shown that scanning 3.75 cm from the central slice in both axial directions (corresponding to a total of 10 additional slices) and 10.5 cm from the center in the radial direction (corresponding to a total of 11 tangential scan lines) results in accurate reconstruction of the 15 cm disk. However, it is evident from the detector response (fig. 1) that the number of additional axial scans required should be increased for objects with a larger diameter in order to allow the number of counts "seen" in these outer slices to be negligible and, hence, not to introduce truncation errors in the 3-D-Fourier transform of the reconstruction. Likewise the number of radial scan lines has to be increased with increasing axial extent of the object to obtain a low number of counts in the line furthest away from the object. These problems are inherent to the scan geometry of the multidetector scanner.

On the multidetector scanner, the patient's shoulders prevent moving the head far enough into the gantry to allow the acquisition of the additional caudal slices required by the 3-D algorithm for an accurate reconstruction of basal slices in the brain. Furthermore, in the radial direction the scanner is limited to distance of 10.5 cm for the scan line furthest away from the patient. These limitations (truncation errors in the projection data) need to be studied further.

Rotating gamma camera

The resolution measured in the center of a water-filled, 20 cm diameter cylindrical phantom using a 128 × 128 matrix format is the same as would be measured for 64 × 64 acquisitions. The MTFs of the projections show that there is no significant under-sampling for the 64 × 64 acquisition [7]. Therefore our resolution measurements can be used in comparisons with the %RMS noise measurements. The lower noise amplification for the windowed reconstructions of the LB collimator (FWHM 1.75 cm) can be translated into an increase in noise-equivalent sensitivity. A reduction of %RMS noise by a factor of 3.1, as observed for the LB collimator at the same number of counts, would required an 9.6 fold increase of the total counts for the LEAP to give the same noise. Even though the LB collimator has a 32% lower count sensitivity than the LEAP, there is still a 3.1 times higher noise-equivalent sensitivity for the LB collimator (with a spatial resolution superior to the LEAP). The advantage of using a high-resolution detector followed by a smoothing process, compared to a low-resolution system without smoothing has long been known in signal processing [9] and has been used for the design of positron tomographs by Phelps [8]. For imaging ^{99m}Tc, a LB collimator of medium-energy design is not favorable for high count sensitivity; however, it has been shown to be advantageous (although not optimized) for the imaging of (p, 2n) ^{123}I with 4–5% contamination by ^{124}I [7].

Our results indicate a great potential for collimators designed for high resolution at even higher sensitivity, for example fan beam geometries [3], matched with an appropriate window in the reconstruction algorithm.

Comparison

A convenient way of comparing SPECT systems would be to measure the image noise for a given resolution in a defined imaging task. Since noise is a function of total counts, the sensitivity for a resolution and slice thickness of 1 cm has been extrapolated by Keyes [2] using an inverse linear relationship between resolution-element volume and sensitivity. This approach, however, does not account for the influence of the reconstruction apodization window on image noise and resolution. We obtained resolution and noise measurements for three combinations of filters, both within the reconstruction plane and in the axial direction. These measurements were then used to predict the noise for scanning a 7.5 cm long, 15 cm diameter cylinder mimicking a brain scan.

First, our measurements on the rotating gamma camera, performed with a 20 cm diameter phantom, were scaled to 15 cm diameter. We use equation (22) introduced by Lim, et al. [4].

$$\%\text{RMS} = K \cdot (A_p/A_c)^{1/2} \cdot D^{3/2} \cdot N_{att}^{-1/2} \cdot f(r)$$

where K is a proportionality constant, A_p the average attenuation in a projection, A_c the attenuation along the diameter of the phantom, D the diameter and N_{att} the attenuated total number of counts in the image. For our calculations we neglected the radial dependence in the noise f(r). N_{att} was computed by numerical integration of all attenuated projection rays over the entire projection. Tab. 3 shows the values of the necessary constants for a 20 cm and 15 cm diameter cylinder with an effective attenuation coefficient of 0.08 cm^{-1}. This coefficient was used rather than 0.14 cm^{-1} to account approximately for the effects of scatter.

Table 3 Constants used to scale noise measured with 20 cm diameter phantom to 15 cm diameter

Phantom diameter	$N_{no\ att}$	N_{att}	$(A_p/A_c)^{1/2}$	$D^{3/2}$
20 cm	314.2	174.4	1.055	89.44
15 cm	176.2	112.1	1.044	58.09

Our measured %RMS noise values, therefore, had to be scaled down by a factor of 0.802 for a 15 cm diameter phantom. We did not account for the improved resolution that would be measured in the smaller phantom; this leads to slight underestimation of the performance of the rotating gamma camera.

As previously described, obtaining ten reconstructed slices of interest (with 0.75 cm spacing) using the multidetector scanner necessitates scanning the object from 20 axial positions. For our simulation of the 7.5 cm-long cylinder, this yielded 52.3×10^6 counts. Scanning 20 slices of the simulated "infinite" cylinder for the same scan time produced 105×10^6 counts. Using the known count sensitivity of the actual scanner for a very long cylinder (12000 cps μCi^{-1} ml), we calculated that this would require 145 minutes scan time. Therefore, the total number of counts expected from scanning 20 overlapped slices of the 7.5 cm long cylinder filled with 1 µCi/ml for 43 minutes is: $(52.3 \times 10^6/145) \times 43 = 15.5 \times 10^6$ counts. Using the measured noise amplification for a thin disk we obtain the predicted %RMS noise in table 2 for our comparison with the gamma camera. We emphasize that these numbers are obtained for data simulated without scatter and attenuation. However, most of the effects of scatter and attenuation on the noise is accounted for by using the measured count sensitivity in the calculation. This assumption seems reasonable since, at least for the rotating gamma camera, $(A_p/A_c)^{1/2}$ in table 3 is close to one. The resolution degradation due to the scatter medium, however, is neglected in our simulation. Therefore, the performance of the multidetector scanner tends to be overestimated.

The analysis described provides three estimates for the image noise for different values of resolution and slice thickness on each SPECT system performing an identical imaging task. Assuming a linear relationship between noise, resolution and slice thickness, we can characterize each system by a plane, defined by the three observations in a 3-dimensional plot of %RMS noise vs. resolution and slice thickness. The origin of our plot (fig. 2) corresponds to zero noise at 1 cm resolution and slice thickness. The plane furthest from the origin (rotating gamma camera with LEAP collimator), describes the poorest performance; the plane closest (multidetector scanner) the best. The approximation that the system performance can be

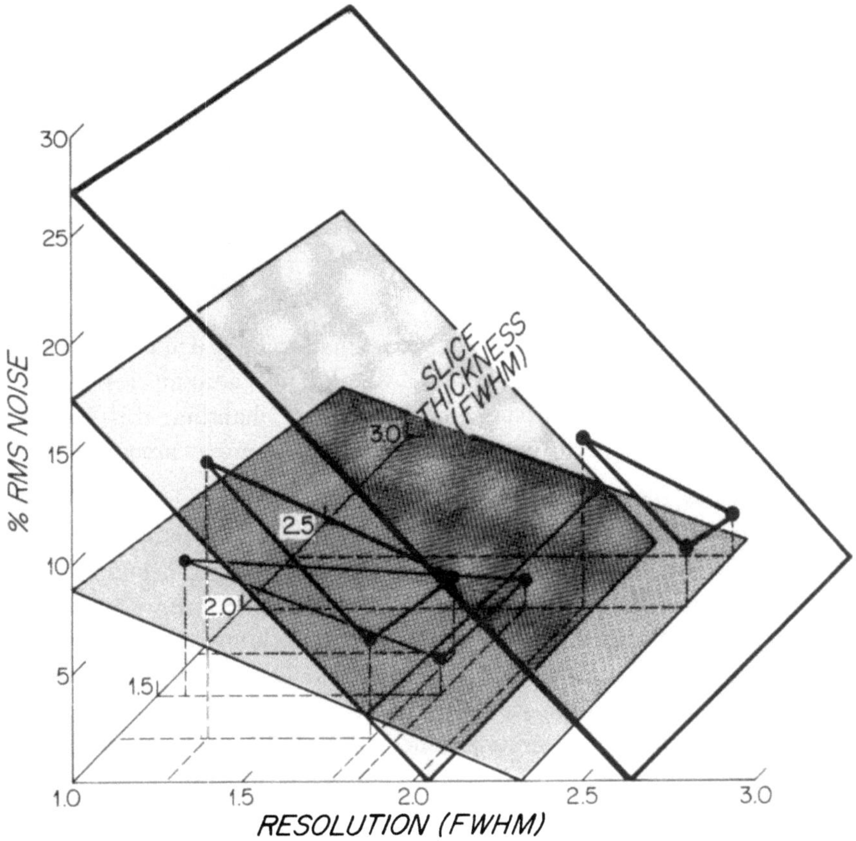

Fig. 2 This 3-D graph shows the relationship between resolution, slice thickness and %RMS noise, predicted for scanning a 7.5 cm long, 15 cm diameter cylindrical phantom (1 μCi/ml) for a total scan time of 43 minutes. For each system, noise, resolution and slice thickness are shown for 3 different combinations of Hanning apodization windows used during reconstruction. These three points define a plane that describes system performance. A plane close to the origin (low noise, good resolution, thin slice) is preferable to a plane further away.

described by a plane is only valid close to the measured data points. The extrapolation to zero noise or zero resolution and slice thickness (neither of which is physically realizable) shows that the plot can be misleading.

The plot confirms our conclusion about the superior performance of the LB vs. the LEAP collimator. Although the multi-detector scanner seems promising, this result should be viewed with caution. In addition to neglecting the effects of scatter and attenuation, the anticipated problems resulting from projection data truncation with a limited axial and radial scan range were not considered and require further investigation.

Acknowledgments

This work was supported in part by grant #1-RO1-N520847 from the Dept. of Health and Human Services, U.S. Public Health Service, Bethesda, Maryland, as well as by a grant from Photon Diagnostics, Inc., Medfield, Massachusetts.

References

[1] Hanson, K.M.: Variations in task and the ideal observer. Proc. SPIE **419** (1983) 60–67.
[2] Keyes, J.W.: Perspectives on tomography, J. Nucl. Med. **23** (1982) 633–640.
[3] Lim, C.B., L.T. Chang, R.J. Jaszczak: Performance analysis of three camera configurations for single photon emission computed tomography. IEEE Tran. Nucl. Sci. NS-**27** (1980) 559–568.
[4] Lim, C.B., S.H. Kyung, E.G. Hawman et al.: Image noise, resolution and lesion detectability in single photon emission CT. IEEE Trans. Nucl. Sci. Ns-**29** (1982) 500–505.
[5] Moore, S.C., M.D. Doherty, R.E. Zimmerman et al.: Improved performance from modifications to the multidetector SPECT brain scanner. J. Nucl. Med. **25** (1984) 688–691.
[6] Moore, S.C., St.P. Mueller: Inversion of the 3-D Radon transform for a multidetector point-focused SPECT brain scanner. Phys. Med. Bio. 31, 1986 (in press).
[7] Mueller, St.P., J.F. Polak, M.F. Kijewski et al.: Performance of SPECT imaging systems: Comparison of a long bore and a LEAP collimator for ^{99m}Tc and ^{123}I. (submitted for publication, 1985).
[8] Phelps, M.E., S.C. Huang, E.J. Hoffman et al.: An analysis of signal amplification using small detectors in positron emission tomography. J. Comp. Assist. Tomogr. **6** (1982) 551–565.
[9] Wagner, R.I.: Decision theory and the detail signal-to-noise ratio of Otto Schade. Phot. Sci. Eng. **22** (1978) 41–46.
[10] Zimmerman, R.E., C.M. Kirsch, R. Lovett et al.: Single photon emission computed tomography with short focal length detectors. In: Single Photon Emission Computed Tomography and other selected Topics, Society of Nuclear Medicine, NY. pp. 148–157, 1980.

IMP SPECT with the Pinhole Collimator

C. Schuemichen, R. Fischer, E. Strauß

Highly sophisticated imaging designs are required to overcome the difficulties in single photon emission tomography. Most problems are still not solved sufficiently. At present time the rotating gamma camera seems to be the most advanced device for this purpose, but even with a double head rotating gamma camera still some problems remain concerning sensitivity, resolution and quantification.

The seven-pinhole collimator tomographic system offers the possibility to perform tomographic scintigraphy using standard nuclear medicine equipment. This technique utilizes a multi-pinhole collimator on a scintillation camera to obtain seven independent, nonoverlapping projections of the organ simultaneously. A computer then reconstructs up to 16 axial tomographic sections. Inherent in this application is quantitative interpretation of the resultant images, utilizing a second computer program.

The seven-pinhole collimator was originally designed by Vogel and co-workers in 1978 [1]. The more pinholes are used, the more axial resolution and sensitivity are gained, but this is parallel to the need of a better intrinsic resolution of the gamma camera. A twelve-pinhole collimator has been the most advanced design in this respect [2]. The seven-pinhole collimator had been available on a commercial base, but was replaced later on by the rotating slant-hole collimator [3].

The seven-pinhole tomography technique has been most successfully aplied to cardiac imaging, application to other organs, such as gated blood pool, thyroid, brain [4]; cisternography, liver [5] and bone has not been really encouraging, at least liver imaging. A suitable collimator design for multi-pinhole brain imaging has not been available commercially.

The purpose of this study was to evaluate the feasibility and utility of the multi-pinhole technique in brain imaging with ^{123}I-amphetamines, using a large field of view seven-pinhole collimator design.

Methods

Performance characteristics of multi-pinhole collimators

In order to understand the difficulties araising from multi-pinhole emission tomography, the imaging performance characteristics of the pinhole is shortly explained.

Planar resolution of the one-pinhole collimator is easily understood. In a standard design, the distance between crystal and pinhole is the same as the effective crystal diameter. Planar resolution Δx, defined as the minimal distance of two pointsources whose images do not overlap, is determined by the intrinsic resolution ε_i of the gamma camera and geometry (tab. 1, fig. 1). Therefore the images should have at least a separation ε_i on the crystal plane. The resolution decreases as one moves away from the pinhole in z-direction.

Table 1 Calculation of resolution

One pinhole planar resolution

$$\Delta X = d + \frac{z}{a} \cdot (d + \varepsilon_i)$$

Seven-Pinhole Emission Tomography

Axial resolution ΔZ: (Z-plane)

$$\Delta Z = Z \cdot \frac{a \cdot \bar{d} + z \cdot (\bar{d} + \varepsilon_i)}{a \cdot c - z \cdot (\bar{d} + \varepsilon_i)}$$

Planar resolution

$$\Delta X = \frac{\Delta Z}{Z + \Delta Z} \cdot (c + \frac{d}{2} \cdot \cos \gamma)$$

Correction for oblique aperture ($\bar{d} \approx d$)

$$\bar{d} = \frac{a \cdot d \cdot \{a \cdot \cos\gamma + \sin\gamma \cdot [\frac{a}{z} \cdot (c - \frac{d}{2} \cos\gamma) - \frac{1}{2} (\varepsilon_i + d \cdot \cos\gamma)]\} + \varepsilon_i \cdot \frac{d^2}{4} \cdot \sin^2\gamma}{a^2 - \frac{d^2}{4} \cdot \sin^2\gamma}$$

a distance crystal – pinhole
d diameter of pinholes
z distance object – pinhole
ε_i intrinsic resolution of the gamma camera (FWHM)
γ angle of obliqueness
c distance of pinholes from center

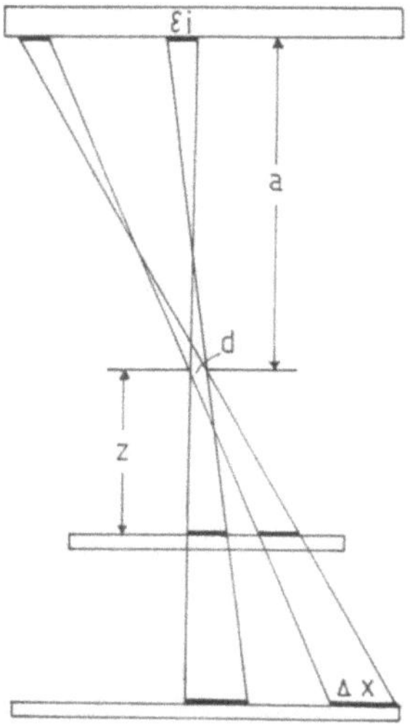

Fig. 1 Planar resolution of the one-pinhole collimator in relation to the distance Z from the pinhole (see also tab. 1).

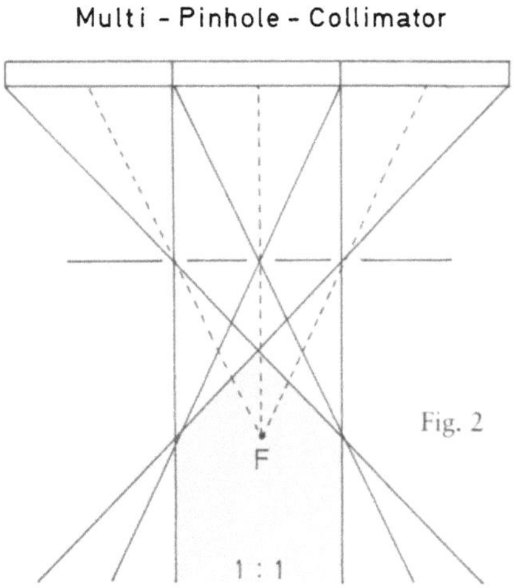

Fig. 2

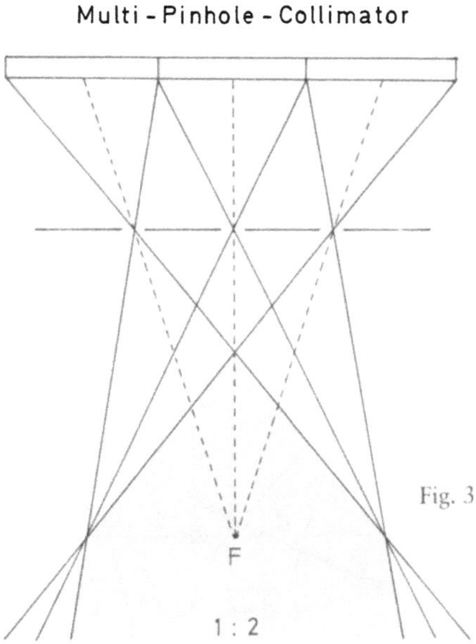

Fig. 3

Fig. 2 Standard design of the seven-pinhole collimator. Distance pinhole plane to focus the same as distance crystal to pinhole plane.

Fig. 3 Large field of view design of the seven-pinhole. Distance pinhole plane to focus twice as much as distance crystal to pinhole plane.

In figures 2 and 3 two different designs of a seven-pinhole collimator are shown, the one in figure 3 represents the standard design. If a large field of view gamma camera with 38 cm effective diameter of the crystal is used, the diameter of each pinhole image will be 12.7 cm. The focus of the collimator shown in figure 2 is in the 12 cm plane from the center pinhole. The second design in figure 3 has a focus af 25.4 cm distance from the center pinhole. If the organ is placed in the focus, it appears in the center of each single image. The field of view in the focus plane is 12 cm for the first and 24 cm for the second design. The first collimator is the standard type for cardiac imaging, the second one may be used for large organs e.g. the brain. However, the imaging performance characteristics of the pinhole in mind, it is evident, that any increase in the field of view will result in a loss of resolution and sensitivity.

Axial resolution was calculated as shown in table 1 and fig. 4. Quantitative data on axial resolution of both collimator designs are shown in tables 2 and 3. Axial means depth in pinhole tomography. The axial resolution depends on the distance of the other pinholes from the center line and on the distance z of the organ from the center pinhole, both together are expressed by the tomographic angle. There is a non-linear relationship between the tomographic angle (or the distance z) and axial resolution.

For the standard collimator design a planar resolution of 1.0 cm and an axial resolution of 1.5 cm in the focus plane was claimed by Vogel and co-workers [1]. Using two point sources we found axial resolution close to the values calculated in tables 2, 3, which represent the worst situation possible. (Picker Dyna Camera 4/37).

In general axial resolution decreases drastically with increasing distance from the pinhole plane, whereas only minor changes in planar (x, y) resolution will occur (tables 2, 3). Below the focus plane axial resolution soon becomes unacceptable. In

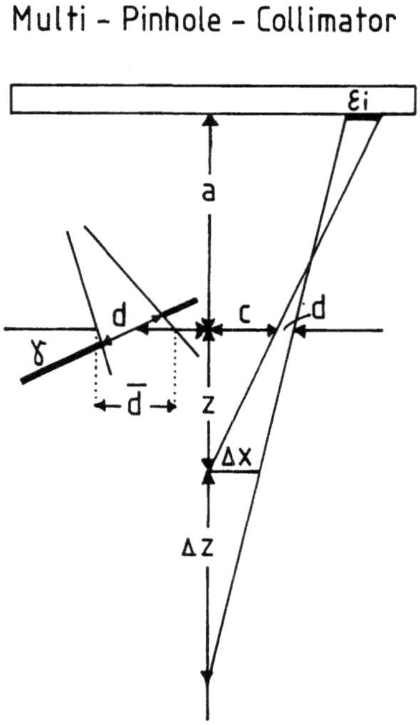

Fig. 4 Planar and axial resolution of the seven-pinhole collimator in relation to the distance Z from the pinhole plane (see also tab. 1).

Table 2 Resolution (FWHM) in seven-pinhole collimator tomography. Standard design. 38 cm gamma camera.
Focus 12,7 cm, field of view at focus plane 12,7 cm, pinhole diameter 0,5 cm, intrinsic resolution of gamma camera 0,5 cm.

Tomographic angle	Plane cm	Axial resolution cm	Planar resolution cm
42.4	7	1.51	1.19
38.7	8	1.82	1.24
35.4	9	2.15	1.29
32.6	10	2.52	1.35
30.2	11	2.93	1.41
28.1	12	3.38	1.47
26.2	13	3.86	1.53
24.6	14	4.39	1.59
23.1	15	4.95	1.65
21.8	16	5.56	1.72
20.6	17	6.22	1.78
19.6	18	6.93	1.85
18.6	19	7.68	1.92
17.7	20	8.49	1.98
16.9	21	9.35	2.05
16.2	22	10.3	2.12
15.5	23	11.2	2.18
14.9	24	12.3	2.25
14.4	25	13.4	2.32

Table 3 Resolution (FWHM) in seven-pinhole collimator tomography. Large field of view design. 38 cm gamma camera. Focus 25,4 cm, field of view at focus plane 25,4 cm, pinhole diameter 0,5 cm, intrinsic resolution of gamma camera 0,5 cm.

Tomographic angle	Plane cm	Axial resolution cm	Planar resolution cm
36.4	11	2.3	1.45
34	12	2.64	1.51
31.9	13	3.01	1.58
30.1	14	3.41	1.64
28.4	15	3.85	1.71
26.9	16	4.31	1.78
25.5	17	4.81	1.84
24.2	18	5.33	1.91
23.1	19	5.9	1.98
22	20	6.5	2.05
21.1	21	7.13	2.12
20.2	22	7.81	2.19
19.4	23	8.52	2.26
18.6	24	9.28	2.33
18	25	10.1	2.4

order to obtain an optimum of resolution the organ has to be placed in the cone above the focus plane. Since here planar resolution exceeds axial resolution, significant blur artifacts occur, that make interpretation of images difficult by inexperienced observers [2]. In the standard collimator design the planar field of view is limited to one third of the effective cristall diameter of the gamma camera. Consequently huge gamma cameras are required for imaging of larger organs. For a given camera size, the planar field of view can be enlarged alternatively by extending the focus of the system. In this case planar resolution remains nearly constant, but an additional decrease of axial resolution and further increase of blur artefacts has to be taken into account.

Collimator design for brain imaging

In combination with a gamma camera with an effective field of view of 38 cm the standard design of the seven-pinhole collimator is suitable for cardiac or thyroid imaging but not for brain imaging. In order to minimize the loss of axial resolution the planar field of view of the brain collimator has to be as large as neccessary but as small as possible. For practical use 20 cm proved to be sufficient. The collimator is shown in fig. 5, its specifications in table 4.

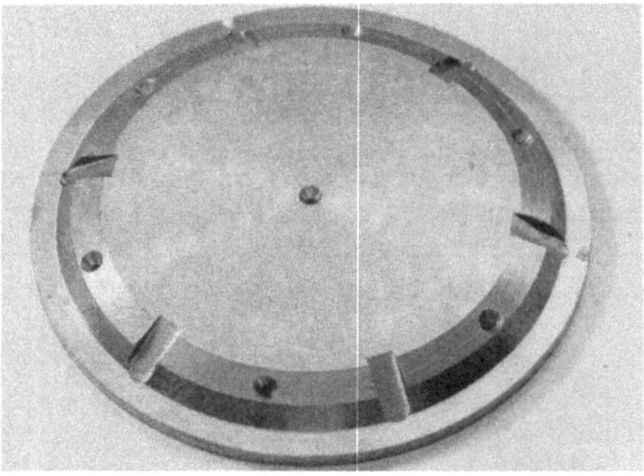

Fig. 5

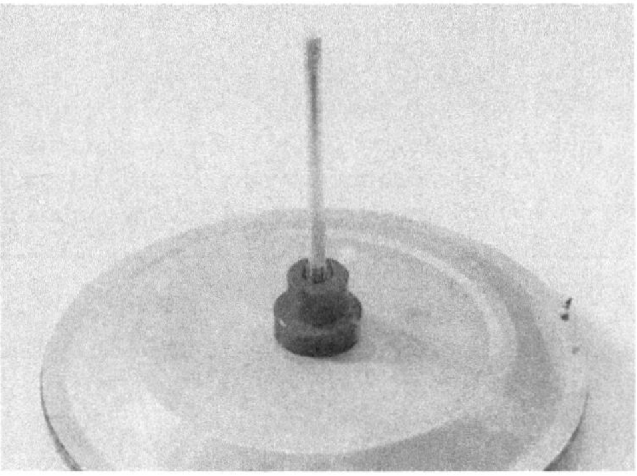

Fig. 6

Fig. 5 Seven-pinhole collimator for brain imaging. Material: high-grade steel.
Fig. 6 Replaceable range-finder on standard seven-pinhole collimator for cardiac imaging.

The normal distance of the collimator surface to the skull is 15 cm, thus only 5 cm depth are left for tomographic imaging with sufficient axial resolution. Under these circumstances patient positioning is even more crucial than it is already in cardiac imaging with the standard seven-pinhole collimator [2]. To make patient positioning more easy, a special range-finder was developed, loosely fixed in the center pinhole of the collimator (fig. 6).

Table 4 Brain collimator design for multi-pinhole tomography

Number of pinholes	7
Distance of pinholes from center	7.7 cm
Diameter of pinholes	0.3 cm
Focus of collimator	20 cm
Planar resolution (FWHM) at focus plane	1.54 cm
Axial resolution (FWHM) at focus plane	4.89 cm
Intrinsic resolution of gamma camera	0.5 cm
Field of view of gamma camera	38 cm
Field of view of collimator at focus plane	20 cm

Results

Brain phantoms studies

A brain phantom was studied, built up with vials, each 2 cm in diameter, lenght 4 cm. The vials were filled with ^{123}I in activity ratios 1.5 : 3 : 5 : 10, simulating the grey and white matter and also hot and cold lesions in both. Results were better than expected from theoretical considerations. Hot and cold lesions could be visualized even in 10 cm depth. However blur artefacts, its origin has been explained, became evident (no figures). Cold lesions at the center of the imaging field, which were reported in literature as artefacts [4], were not observed.

Static brain imaging

Static imaging was done routinely in three projections (axial, frontal, posterior) between 60 and 90 minutes after application of 5 mCi ^{123}I-amphetamine (without ^{124}I contamination). In all projections the grey and white method was clearly deliniated, but difficulties arose in vizualization of the brain stem and cerebellum (fig. 7 a–d).

Dynamic brain imaging

Because of the relative high sensitivity of the seven-pinhole collimator tomographic system and because of the lack of any detector movement the ability of dynamic sequence imaging is offered.

Imaging in axial position was started immediately after application of 5 mCi ^{123}I-amphetamine. 60 sequences of one minute duration were recorded. For documenta-

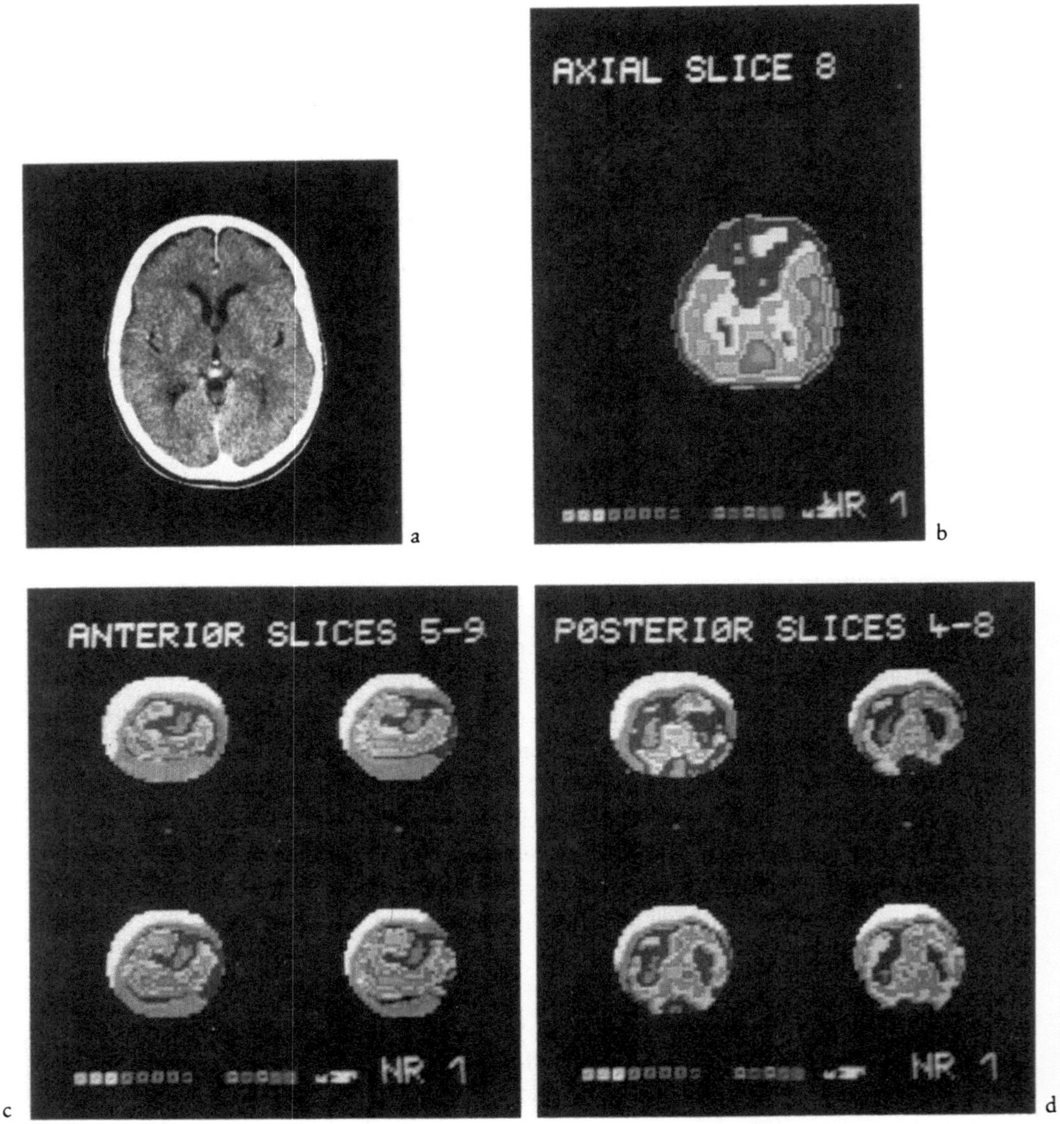

Fig. 7 58 years old female patient with TIA. IMP SPECT with seven-pinhole collimator showed decreased uptake in left hemisphere.
a) Axial CT, normal; b) Axial SPECT, brain-stem not clearly seen even on deeper cuts; c) Anterior SPECT; d) Posterior SPECT, cerebellum not seen even on deeper cuts.

tion 5–10 sequences were summarized to one image. One example is shown in fig. 8 a, b.

Initial perfusion (1–5 minutes p.i.) of the left front lobe appeared normal, whereas uptake of ^{123}I-amphetamine in this area later on (50–60 min p.i.) was low. Delayed imaging (6 h p.i.) showed a significant redistribution of the tracer in this area, indicating the presence of vital brain tissue.

a 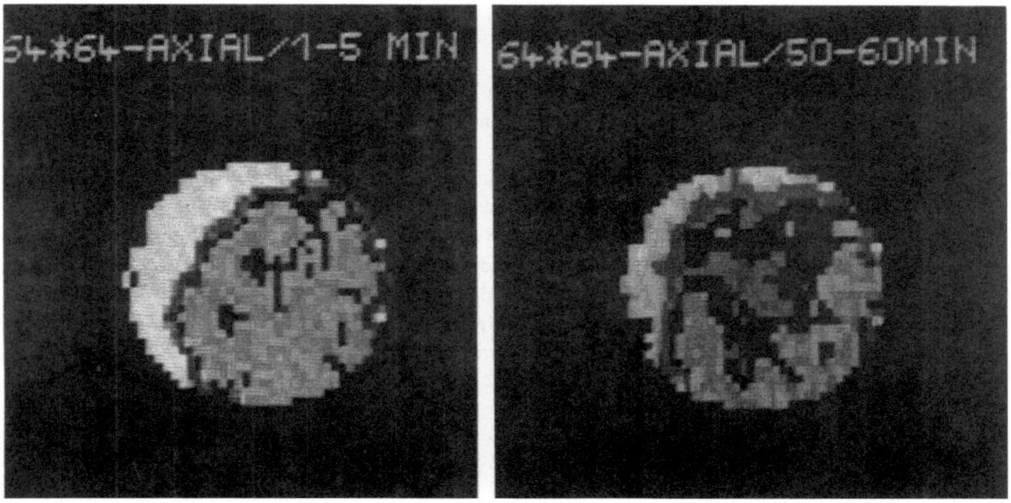 b

Fig. 8 62 year old male patient with infarction left front lobe. Axial IMP SPECT
a) Perfusion image 1–5 min p.i. Normal perfusion in left front lobe; b) Delayed image 50–60 min. p.i. Decreased uptake in left front-lobe despite normal initial perfusion.

Conclusions

Despite certain drawbacks of low angle tomography, such as poor depth resolution, the seven-pinhole tomography system provides new imaging modalities, not feasable with rotating systems. Brain imaging with ^{123}I-amphetamine will benefit by dynamic imaging in obtaining basic information about brain perfusion, not available by other tomographic systems.

Summary

Low angle tomography with the seven-pinhole collimator system is characterized by a sufficient sensitivity and the lack of detector movement. For brain imaging the tomographic angle must be kept low to obtain a sufficient large field of view. By this axial resolution is considerably lower than planar resolution, the brain-stem and the cerebellum are not visualized clearly and blur-artefacts are no longer negligable. On the other hand the system offers the ability of dynamic sequence imaging. Evaluation of the initial perfusion in areas with low uptake of ^{123}I-amphetamine later on provides additional information about the vitality of this tissue without the need of delayed imaging.

References

[1] Vogel, R. A., D. L. Kirch, M. T. Lefree et al.: A New Method of Multiplanar Emission Tomography. Using a Seven Pinhole Collimator and an Anger Scintillation Camera. J. Nucl. Med. **19** (1978) 648–654.

[2] Kirch, D. L., B. Hasegawa, D. Stern et al.: An Improved Twelve-Pinhole System for Emission Cardiac Tomography. J. Nucl. Med. **22** (1981) P33 (abst.).

[3] Lewis, S. E., E. M. Stokely, M. D. Devous, S. R. et al.: Quantitation of Experimental Canine Infarct Size with Multipinhole and Rotating-Slanthole Tomography. J. Nucl. Med. **22** (1981) 1000–1005.

[4] Grove, R. B., A. Rodewald, R. L. Bell et al.: Application of Multiple Pinhole Emission Radionuclide Tomography to Imaging of the Brain and Thyroid. J. Nucl. Med. **22** (1981) P87 (abst.).

[5] Chang, W., S. L. Lin, R. E. Henkin: A Study Demonstrating that the Heart is the Only Suitable Organ for Collimator Tomography. J. Nucl. Med. **22** (1981) P34 (abst.).

II Clinical Results

Clinical Relevance of N-Isopropyl-(^{123}I)p-Iodoamphetamine (IMP) SPECT Brain Imaging

I. Podreka, K. Höll, P. Dal Bianco, G. Goldenberg, D. Wimberger, E. Auff, Th. Brücke

Summary

SPECT studies of the brain were performed by means of N-isopropyl-(^{123}I)p-iodoamphetamine and a double head rotating scintillation camera. Energy spectra showed an increase of scattered radiation proportional to the geometrical resolution of the used Tc-collimators. This is due to the higher lead content and thin septa (septum-penetration of high energy photons of ^{123}I, scattering in the crystal) of HRES or UHRES collimators. A LEAP collimator (14 mm FWHM resolution in the reconstructed image) is the most suitable one (sufficient resolution – relatively low scatter-fraction) for ^{123}I labeled tracers. With a multiple window technique scatter correction was performed. The width and position of the scatter windows were estimated in phantom studies. Further steps of data processing (prereconstructional filtering, analytical attenuation compensation), leading to an improvement of the final set of cross sections, are described. Clinical cases (Alzheimers, Huntingtons, Parkinsons disease, Moya Moya, stroke and partial complex seizures) and stimulation (acoustic memory tasks, visual stimulations) studies in normal volunteers are presented, and results are compared with PET-data known from recent literature.

Introduction

Since the development of N-isopropyl-(^{123}I)p-iodoamphetamine by Winchell et al. [1, 2], several reports concerning the clinical application of this compound have been published. Mainly, IMP studies have been performed in stroke [3, 4] or epilepsy [5, 6] showing decreased IMP uptake in the ischemic area or epileptogenic focus. Unfortunately, the obtained SPECT images are usually of poor quality, due to several physical factors, no matter if a multidetector device or a scintillation camera is used. Thus, the resolution and statistic accuracy of PET images has never been reached. Concerning these severe drawbacks, it is questionable if SPECT can become an important tool in daily clinical routine.

The purpose of this paper is first to show how SPECT-brain imaging can be improved by adequate image processing and second to compare obtained results in several neurological disorders with PET-data known from recent literature.

Methods

System Description

In our institute, SPECT is performed with a dual head rotating scintillation camera (SIEMENS ZLC37), which is connected to a computer system (NODECREST MICAS2000). The patient is placed in supine position on a dentist's chair, the head is fixed in a thin cylindrical plastic head holder, and therefore the organ of interest extends only to the lower half of the camera field. The detectors can clear the shoulders, so the diameter of rotation can be reduced to 250 mm in order to

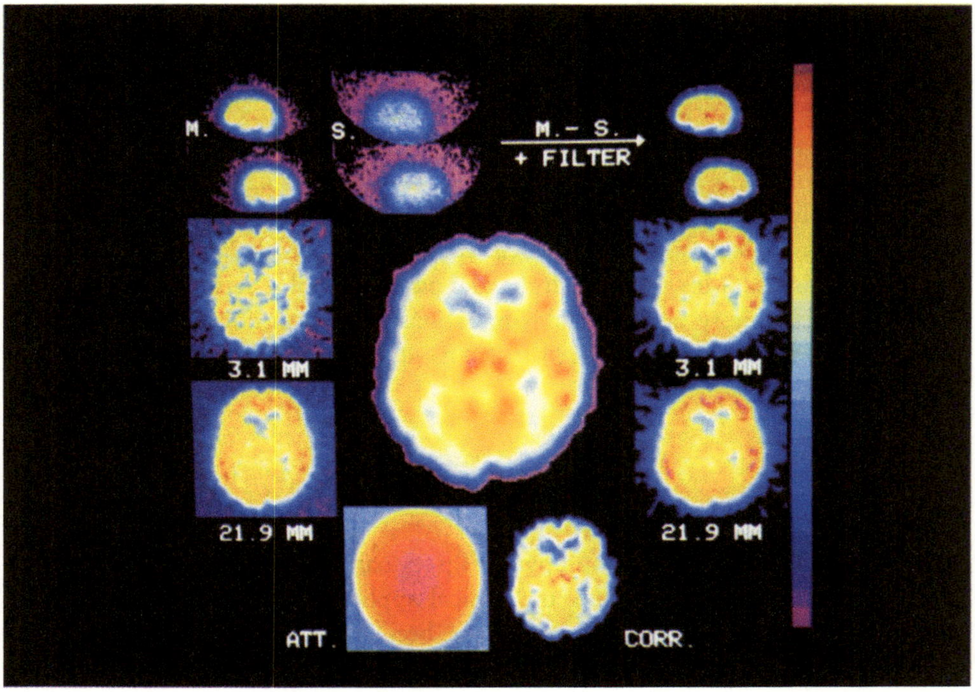

Fig. 1 The different steps of data processing are summarized. One pair of projection-data registered in the main and in the scatter windows are shown. After the subtraction, projections are filtered to improve signal-to-noise ratio. Then, elliptic boundaries are defined on each single slice, to correct projections for attenuation. Consecutive summation of 7 single slices leads to the final, quantitatively relevant cross section (centre of fig.).

improve scanning conditions. 30 min. after i.v. administration of 6–6.5 mCi ^{123}I (produced by the p,5n reaction and free of ^{124}I), 60 (2 × 30) projections (100 sec/angle, linear sampling distance of 3.125 mm) are recorded.

After scatter correction, the projection image set is filtered with a weighted-smooth filter of variable shape and size [7] to supress noise. By reorganisation of the corrected projections, a sinogram is created and 3.125 mm thick horizontal slices are reconstructed by filtered backprojection [8] in 128 × 128 matrices. Then, each slice is corrected for tissue absorption following the model of Bellini et al. [9]. 8 transversal slices are summed consecutively to give a set of 21.9 mm thick, quantitatively relevant [10] cross sections covering the whole organ for final evaluation of the study. The resolution in one slice is 14 mm FWHM (line source in scatter medium), and each slice contains 300.000–350.000 cts (fig. 1).

Scatter Correction and Choice of Collimators

2.5–3% of the decay of ^{123}I occurs in radiation of 350–550 keV. These high energy photons penetrate the septa of Tc-collimators and scatter in the crystal itself [11], which leads to an increase of noise over the entire energy spectrum. Therefore, an asymetrical energy window allows only imperfect discrimination against scattered photons [12]. Fig. 2 displays energy spectra of ^{123}I obtained with HSENS, LEAP and HRES Tc-collimators. The increase of the scatter fraction is directly proportional to the lead content of the collimator; thus, increasing the geometrical resolution leads to decreasing energy resolution.

For the estimation of the scatter fraction recorded in the main energy window (159 keV ± 10%), an empirical procedure was employed. First, a Hoffmans brain phantom (fig. 3) was filled with ^{99m}Tc and scanned at 100 mm distance to function as a reference. Since it is possible to use 3 different energy windows simultanously, an additional window was set on each side of the main in experiments with ^{123}I. The width and position of the "scatter"-windows were varied, and corrected pixel contents were compared with the Tc-reference. Minimum difference in % was found when windows were set at 142 keV ± 6% and 177 keV ± 5%. Fig. 3 shows the improvement in ^{123}I image contrast after scatter subtraction. In order to simulate patient conditions, experiments were repeated with a skull-phantom with plastic ventricles (cold lesion). With the proposed windows, the ^{123}I cross sectional matrices gave nearly the same pixel values as the ^{99m}Tc-study. The scatter fraction registered in the main-peak window was found to be appr. 38% for the LEAP collimator, 50% for the HRES and 65% for the UHRES. Thus, only LEAP collimators which still have relevant resolution are the only suitable ones for IMP-SPECT imaging of the brain.

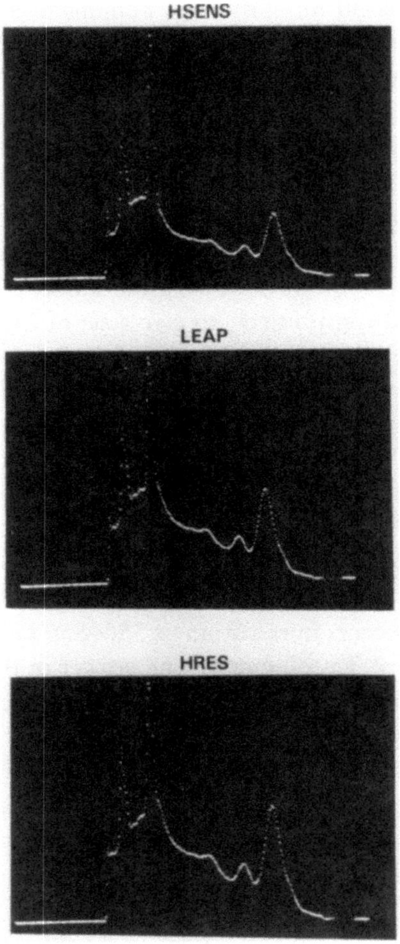

Fig. 2 Energy spectra obtained with different Tc-collimators, demonstrating a significant increase of the high energy secondary peak whose Compton part superposes the entire energy spectrum. This increase of the secondary peak is directly proportional to the lead content of the collimators. Thus, increasing geometrical resolution leads to decreasing energy resolution.

Clinical studies

370 IMP-SPECT studies have been carried out since 1983. Patients suffering from stroke, epilepsy, Huntingtons and Parkinsons diseases and shizophrenia were investigated. Furthermore, neuropsychological studies were performed on normal volunteers (who gave informed consent) during different acoustic memory tasks and visual stimulation. It is, however, beyond the scope of this paper to present all obtained results; instead, we will concentrate on individual clinical cases which exhibit abnormalities in IMP distribution similar to those obtained by FDG-PET. In addition, stimulation studies will be shown. Furthermore, the identifying of brain

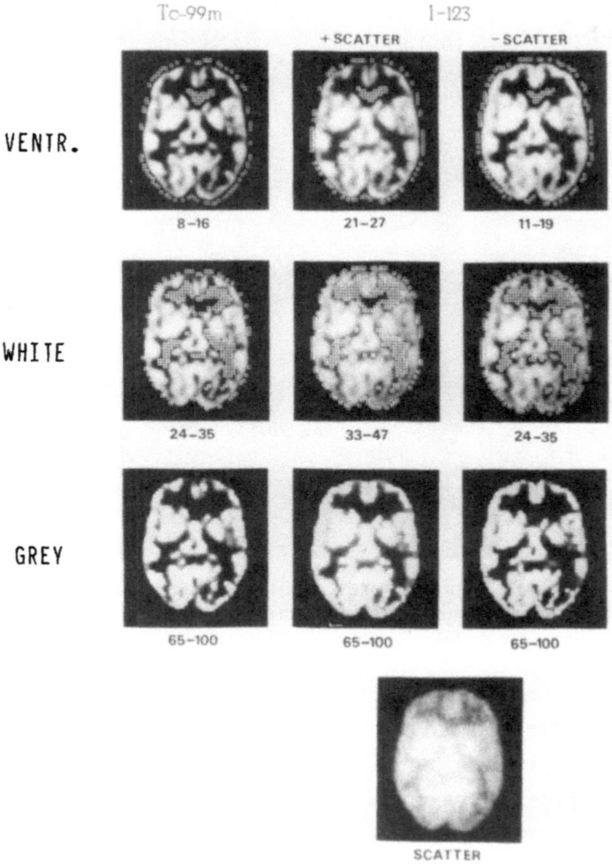

Fig. 3 Left (^{99m}Tc) column and middle (^{123}I) show planar images of Hoffmans phantom. The figures are related to the activity content of the respective regions (% of maximum). The right column shows the results of the proposed scatter correction (note minimum difference to the Tc-study), lower right is the scatter image.

structures was standardized by comparing the SPECT images with cross-section image sets of "An Atlas of the Human Brain for Computerized Tomography" [13].

Resting state: B. H., f, 40 a (right-handed normal volunteer). IMP study was performed during resting state (darkened room and low background noise). Good differentiation of cortical and subcortical structures was obtained. The following distributions of IMP in % of maximum brain isotope uptake (fig. 4) were recorded:

90–100%: superior frontal and cingulate gyri, superior parts of occipital lobes, thalami

80– 89%: superior and inferior frontal gyri, superior temporal lobes, anterior basal ganglia, thalami, brain stem and cerebellum

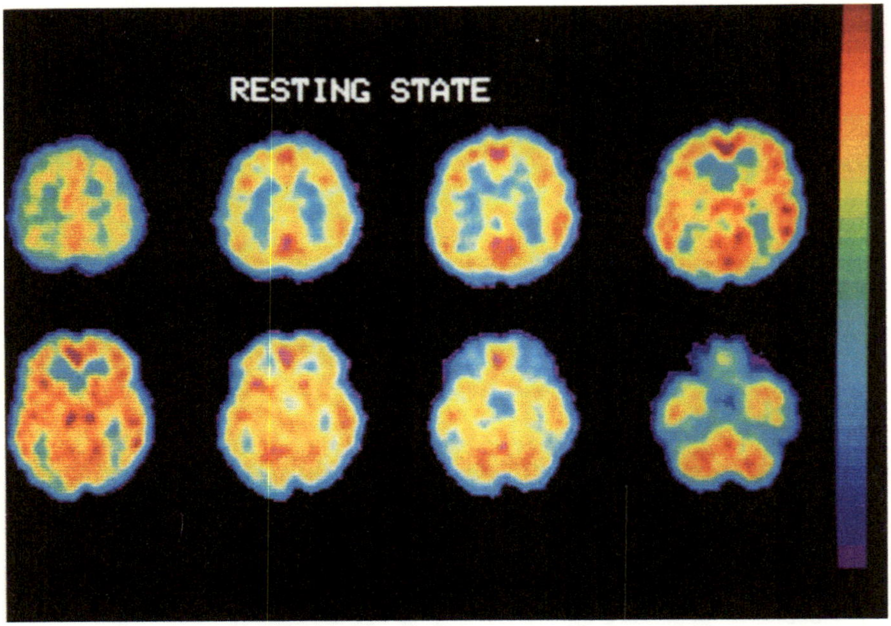

Fig. 4 Resting state: Symetric IMP-distribution with highest tracer-uptake in the frontal and occipital lobes, thalami, the caudate-putamen complex and cerebellum.

70– 79%: superior frontal and middle frontal gyri, paracentral lobule, temporal lobes, hypocampus, cerebellum
65– 69%: parietal lobe, inferior temporal gyri
50– 64%: boundary pixels between gray and white matter
40– 49%: white matter and ventricles in part
30– 39%: ventricles in part, chiasmatic cistern
20– 29%: chiasmatic cistern

Thus, highest rCBF values were found in the frontal and occipital lobes, thalami, the caudate-putamen complex, and cerebellum, which correlate to PET data [14].

Alzheimers disease: B. H., f, 62 a suffered of progredient dementia for appr. 1 year. Disorientation for place and time, severe deficits of higher cerebral functions, especially of verbal and visual memory were present. CT-scan revealed cortical atrophy, while IMP-SPECT showed low uptake of the tracer in parieto-temporal regions and left frontal lobe. The distribution pattern of the tracer corresponds to metabolic images in Alzheimers disease [15] (fig. 5).

Disorders of the extrapyramidal system

Huntingtons disease: P. M., m, 35 a showed typical symptoms of this disease for 3 years. Psychoorganic syndrome was present. CT-scan showed enlargement of ventricles and atrophic cortical changes. In IMP-SPECT no deposition of the tracer

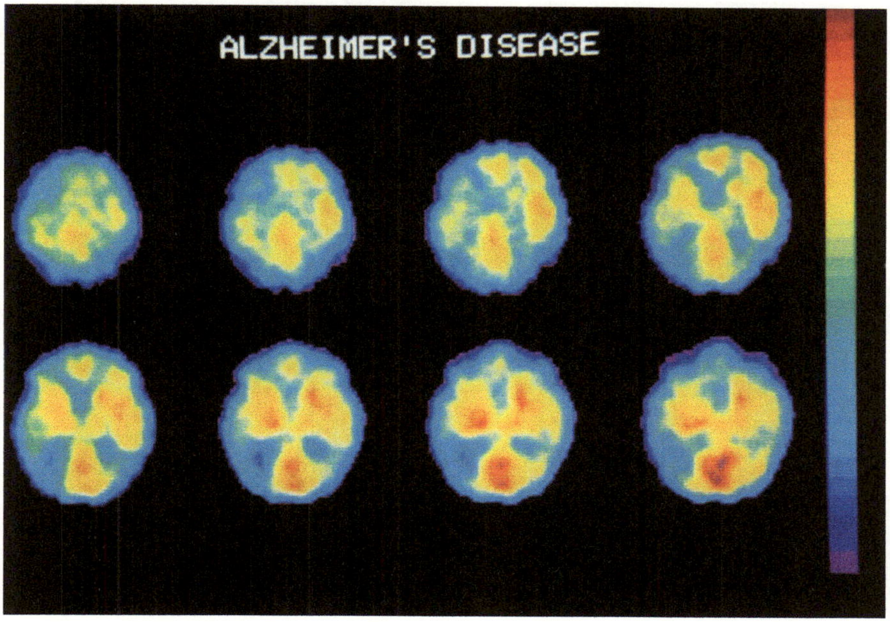

Fig. 5 Alzheimer's disease: SPECT shows decreased IMP-uptake in the left frontal lobe and in both parieto-temporal regions corresponding to metabolic images.

was seen in the anterior basal ganglia. IMP-uptake was low in the thalami and in both parietal lobes (fig. 6).

Hemiparkinsonism: L. L., f, 45 a. For 1½ years this patient has developed slight rigidity, gait disturbance and left-sided tremor of the upper and lower limbs. Signs of dementia were absent. Medication with L-DOPA led to improvement of clinical symptoms. CT-scan was normal. The IMP study demonstrates lower IMP uptake in the right anterior basal ganglia and thalamus than on the left side (fig. 7).

Cerebrovascular disorders

Moya Moya: Z. H., m, 52 a. Typical angiographic patterns for this disease were found in this patient. No hemiparesis, but an psychoorganic syndrome was present. The result of CT-scan is unknown. IMP-SPECT showed ischemic areas in both frontal lobes, which were more pronounced on the left side, right insula and in the right inferior occipital cortex (fig. 8).

Stroke: W. L., f, 43 a. Three months prior to admission, she had an ischemic stroke with left-sided hemiparesis. Neurological symptoms resolved nearly completely after two weeks. At time of SPECT only leftsided accentuation of reflexes and positive pyramidal signs were present. CT-scan showed a hypodense lesion in the anterior part of the internal capsula extending to the right putamen. IMP study revealed,

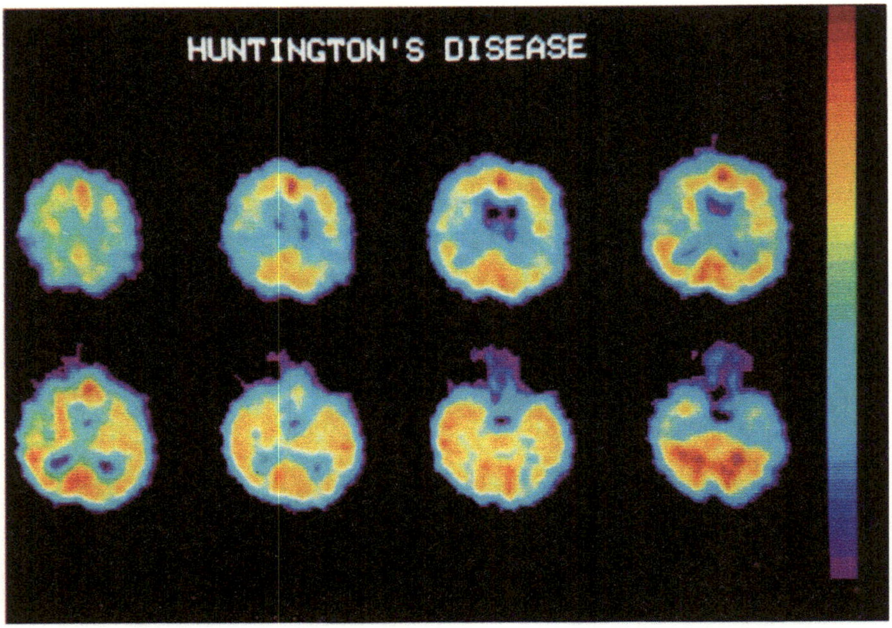

Fig. 6 Huntingtons disease: IMP-SPECT reveals no tracer-uptake in the anterior basal ganglia, low in the thalami and in both parietal lobes.

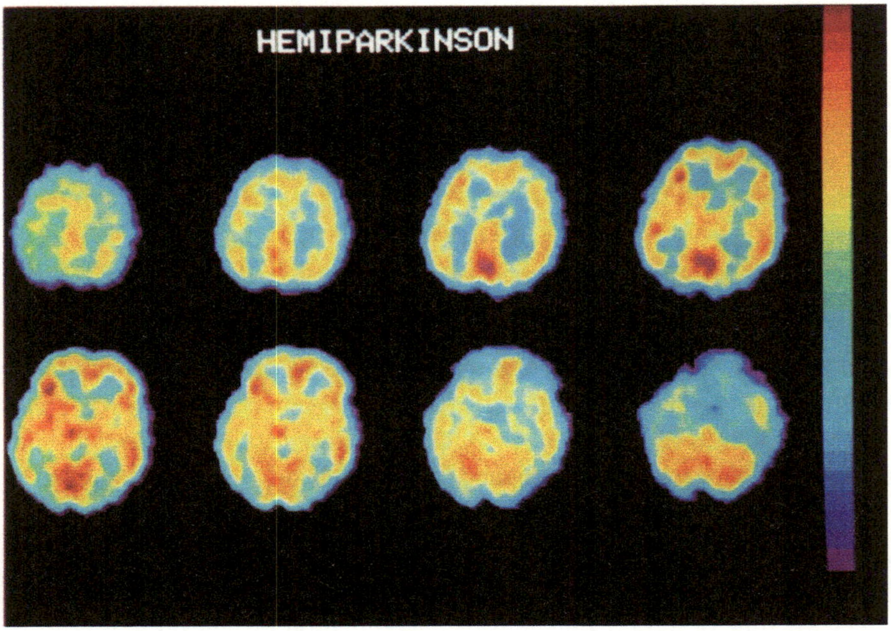

Fig. 7 Hemiparkinsonism: Note lower IMP-uptake in the right anterior basal ganglia and thalamus than on the left side.

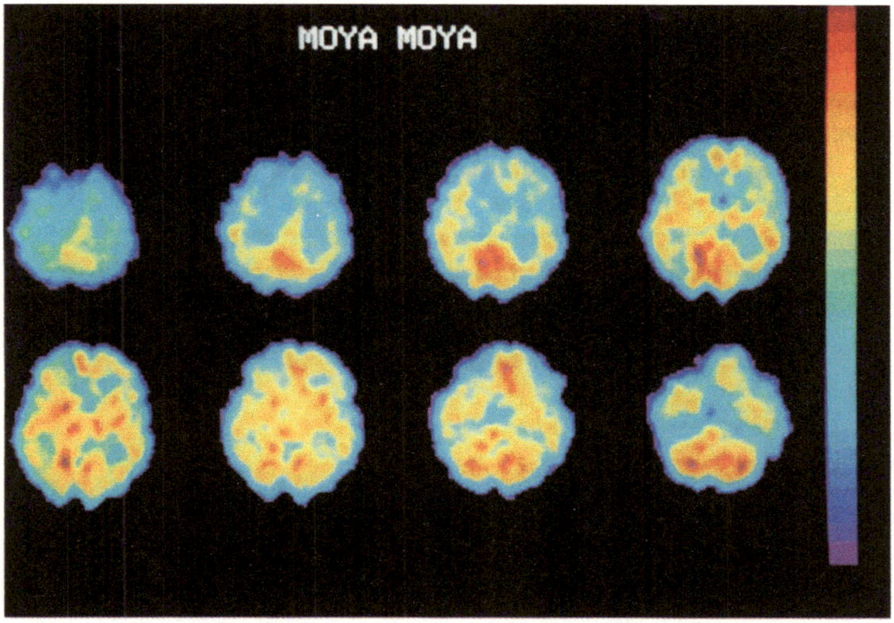

Fig. 8 Moya Moya: IMP-SPECT demonstrates ischemic areas in both frontal lobes (more pronounced on the left side), right insula and in the right inferior occipital cortex.

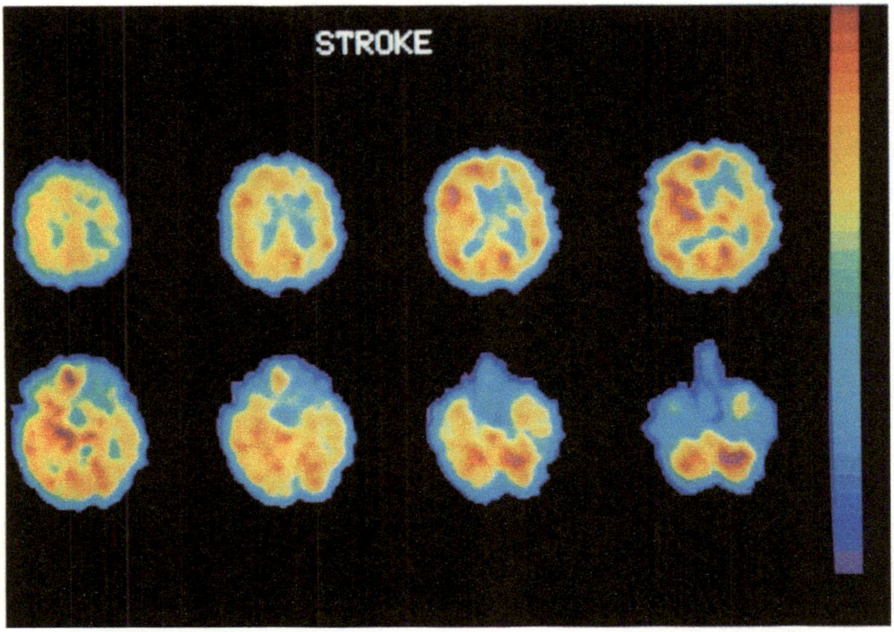

Fig. 9 Stroke: CT-scan showed a hypodense lesion in the anterior part of the internal capsula extending to the right putamen. IMP-SPECT study demonstrates the lesion in the same location and distribution as CT-scan. In addition, there is deactivation of the right frontal lobe and crossed cerebellar diaschisis.

besides the lesion visible on CT, deactivation of the right frontal lobe and crossed-cerebellar diaschisis (fig. 9).

Partial complex seizures: G. W., m, 30 a had, one year prior to investigation, one tonic-clonic seizure. Three days before SPECT a partial complex seizure was observed. He was having his breakfast and suddenly heard far voices. In state of impaired consciousness he walked naked through town for one hour and was then brought home. EEG revealed a left temporal focus, CT-scan was normal. SPECT showed in seizure-free state a decreased deposition of tracer in the left middle temporal gyrus, while in the left superior temporal lobe increased IMP uptake was observed. A control study six months later showed the same isotope distribution (fig. 10).

Stimulation studies

Different acoustic memory tasks were performed. Here two studies are shown:

SCH. G., f, 21 a, right-handed was listening via earphones to a list of concrete nouns. She was instructed to memorize the words and to switch a lamp if repetition occured. Her eyes were blindfolded. Under this condition increased IMP deposition occurred in both superior frontal gyri, both medial frontal regions, right inferior parietal area and both superior temporal gyri. (fig. 11)

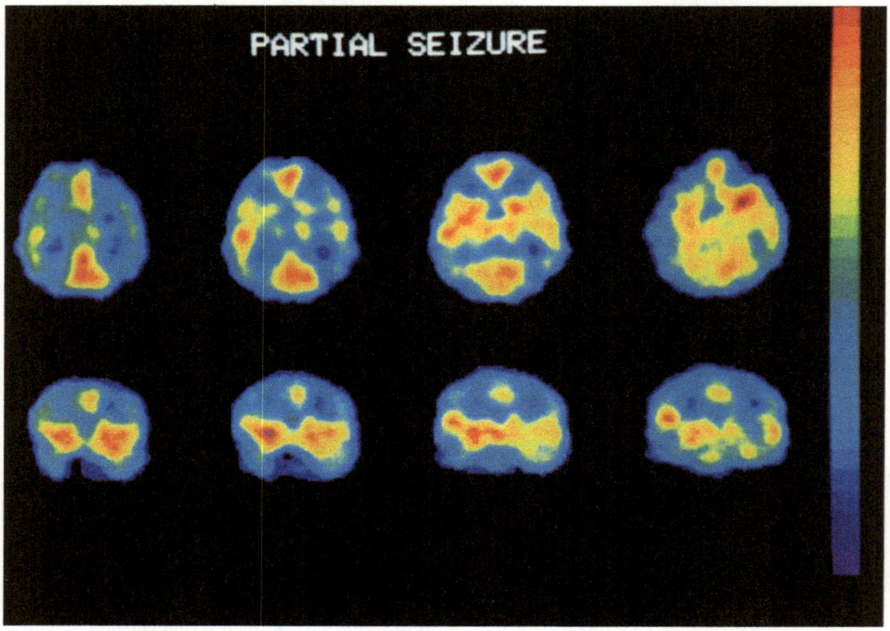

Fig. 10 Partial complex seizures: Axial and coronar slices show decreased IMP-deposition in the left middle and inferior temporal gyrus, while IMP-uptake in the left superior temporal gyrus is increased.

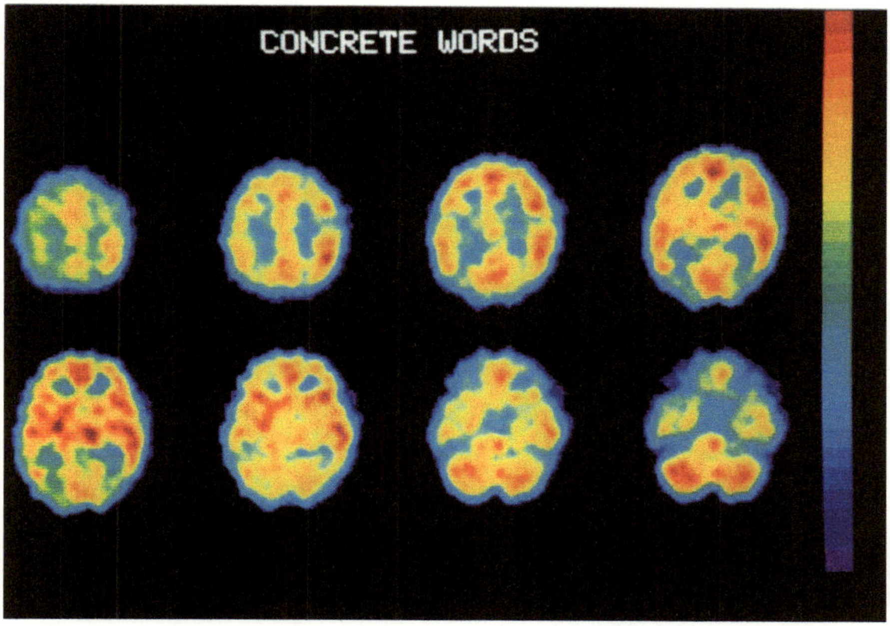

Fig. 11 Acoustic stimulation: of a normal right-handed volunteer. Memorizing concrete nouns led to increased IMP-deposition in both superior frontal gyri, both medial frontal regions, right inferior parietal area and both superior temporal gyri.

B. H., m, 24 a, right-handed performed the same task, but had to employ visual imagery to solve the task. Activation of both superior frontal regions, left medial frontal gyrus, left interior frontal region, both superior temporal regions (more pronounced on the left) and both occipital lobes was observed, while the inferior part of the visual cortex was activated only on the left side (fig. 12).

Visual stimulation was performed with a pair of diode-spectacles using a frequency of 1.5/sec and intensity of 400 mcD/m^2. During SPECT VEP were recorded. In a 27 years old normal volunteer, activation in both visual cortices was seen (fig. 13a), while in a patient (41 a, f) suffering from chorioretinitis pigmentosa, no increase, but lower IMP deposition as compared to normal resting state was found in the visual cortex (fig. 13b). This patient's visual potentials could not be evoked.

(Activation patterns were derived by comparison of IMP distributions between a resting state group (n = 14) and different task groups [16].)

Discussion

Emission computerizied tomography (ECT) of the brain is designed to evidence and evaluate quantitatively cerebral blood flow and metabolic processes. With this technique, isotope distribution in deep brain structures, such as basal ganglia, can be detected and artifacts in quantitation avoided (e.g., the superposition of different

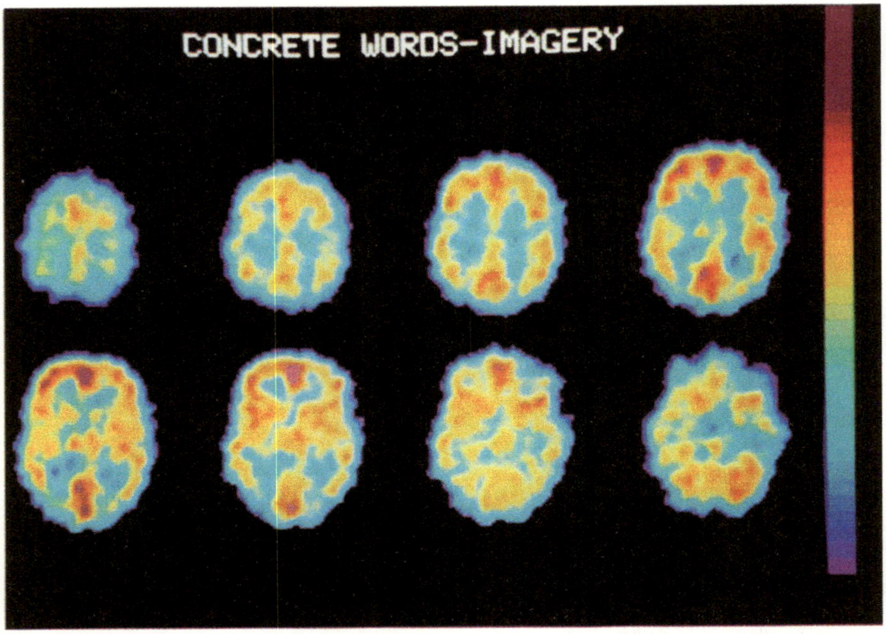

Fig. 12 IMP-SPECT study of a normal right-handed volunteer, who had to employ his imagery during memorizing concrete nouns. Activation is seen in both superior frontal regions, left medial frontal gyrus, left inferior frontal region, both superior temporal regions (more pronounced on the left side), and both occipital lobes. Note that the inferior part of the visual cortex is activated only on the left side.

tissue components [17], or "cross talk" from one hemisphere [18] as it is common in two dimensional techniques).

The application of positron emission tomography (PET) in neurology has opened new dimensions in understanding the nature of pathological processes in several diseases affecting the central nervous system. PET studies have been done in normal aging [19, 20], stroke [21–23], epilepsy [24–27], Huntingtons and Parkinsons disease [28–30], and various forms of dementia [31]. Furthermore, specific binding sites as dopamine- [32, 33] or opiate- [34] receptors and activation of brain regions during specific stimulations [35, 36] have been visualized.

The quantitative analysis of such investigations offers the possibility to speculate on the development and progression of neurological disorders, and it will lead to new concepts of disease mechanism and cognitive networks.

However, the complexity of PET and the cost of this cyclotron-based technology limit access to few institutes. Single photon emission computerized tomography (SPECT) can be performed with special multidetector devices or commercially available rotating gamma cameras at relatively low cost. Despite the high sensitivity of SPECT-multidetector devices [37–39], the resolution of which is comparable to elder PET systems, the obtained images show usually low or equivocal distinction of brain structures due to blurring-artifacts and poor contrast.

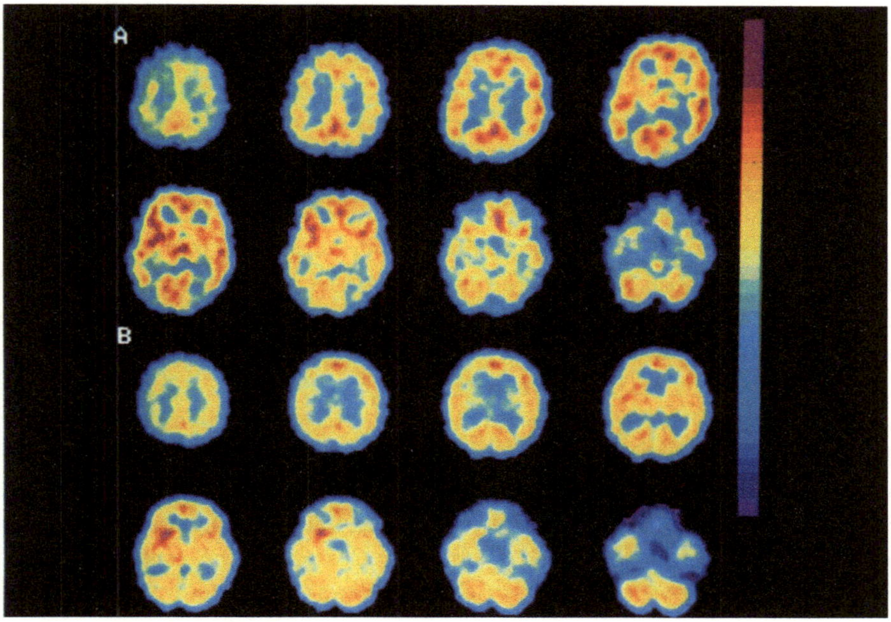

Fig. 13 Visual stimulation of (a) a normal individual. IMP-SPECT shows activation in both visual cortices. Whereas, in a case of chorioretinitis pigmentosa (b), no increase, but lower IMP-deposition as compared to normal resting state was found in the visual cortex. Both sets of images correlate with VEP results.

Besides accurate system performance, adequate image processing is substantial for the quality of SPECT images. We believe we have been able to reach reasonable resolution and sufficient contrast in our images. This improvement is based on:

a) reduction of diameter of rotation to 250 mm without modifications of the camera [40] or utilization of slant hole collimators [41], but only by changing the patients support (dentist's chair) and costructing a thin plastic head holder
b) uniformity of the scintillation camera (ZLC system)
c) employment of LEAP collimators in order to get reasonable counting rates, resolution, and tolerable scatter fraction for IMP-brain SPECT.
d) extension of scanning time to 50 min. Appr. 10 mill. cts are recorded in normal subjects. After scatter subtraction one final cross section contains 300.000–350.000 cts.
e) prereconstructional multiple window scatter correction [12] and proper energy window setting followed by sensitivity control prior to each patient study
f) filtering of the projection image set (in order to enhance contrast and suppress Poisson noise [42, 43] without losing resolution) with a weighted smooth filter of variable shape and size [44] prior to reconstruction
g) linear sampling distance of 3.125 mm, reconstruction in 128 × 128 matrices, and analytical attenuation correction of each 3.125 mm thick slice [9]

This complex data handling leads to SPECT images with good distinction of gray and white matter (ratio = 2.2) in 21.9 mm slices, brain lobes – particularly of the visual cortex, thalamus and anterior basal ganglia, as well as of the brain stem and the cerebellum (fig. 4). Analysing the full set of cross sections, adequate information about isotope distribution in the brain is obtained, even if the cross-sectional plane is not parallel to the orbito-meatal line.

Thus, IMP-SPECT becomes a feasible clinical tool in recognising pathologic processes of various neurological disorders. From our experience epileptogenic foci could be detected in 72% of patients with partial seizures and normal CT-scan; in some instances hyperperfused areas adjacent to regions with low CBF were seen interictally. These results correlate with several PET findings [24, 25, 27, 45]. As has been demonstrated, deactivation of noninfarcted brain tissue and crossed cerebellar diaschisis can be evidenced. Also, disorders involving the extrapyramidal system can be recognized in IMP-SPECT. Furthermore, it is possible to perform investigations on brain organisation during specific stimulations. Extended clinical and neuropsychological studies can be performed in many nuclear medicine centres and will confirm PET research.

Several sources of error, however, are inherent to ECT: inadequate kinetic models, improper system performance, inaccurate scatter- or attenuation correction, deficient image processing or reconstruction algorithms, erroneus identification of brain structures, but also the partial volume effect, can severely distort quantitative data. Opinions on the absolute quantitation of IMP-SPECT are controversial due to not fully elucidated IMP kinetics. Kuhl et al. [46, 47] have shown good correlations between rCBF values obtained with microspheres and IMP in dogs. In humans stable cortex/white-matter-activity ratios were found throughout the first hour after isotope injection, and it was proposed that also "1h-images" could be quantified. Other authors [48, 49] described changes in IMP uptake in infarcted tissue 5h after tracer administration. If this redistribution exists already within the first two hours, quantitation would not be possible. We could see in one stroke patient "luxury perfusion" five days after the insult, while 14 days later the control study revealed decreased IMP deposition in the infarcted area, corresponding to the persistence of hemiparesis. Repeated scanning in other two stroke patients did not show redistribution of the tracer between 30–150 min. in the ischemic region.

We have evidence (unpublished data) that rCBF values are reproducible in normal subjects using the microsphere model [47] and its correction for individual 0–5 min IMP inflow of "stable" IMP images (30–80 min. after bolus) [50]. If quantitation in SPECT is considered, however, the problem of methodological errors arises. Despite good resolution, small variations in isotope distribution during acquisition or improper blood sampling lead to fluctuations of rCBF values. When ^{133}Xe is used for estimation of rCBF, fluctuations of the input function (improper breathing of the patient) or poorly resolved brain structures [51, 52] (although high dosages (70–200 mCi) are administrated) affect seriously rCBF values [53, 54], and furthermore the partition coefficient of ^{133}Xe in ischemic tissue is unknown. Future clinical application will show, if quantitation of SPECT-studies will give reliable results.

References

[1] Winchell, H. S., W. D. Horst, L. Braun et a.: N-Isopropyl-(^{123}I)p-Iodoamphetamine: single-pass brain uptake and washout; binding to the brain synaptosomes; and localization in dog and monkey brain. J. Nucl. Med. **21** (1980) 947–952.

[2] Winchell, H. S., R. M. Baldwin, T. H. Lin: Development of ^{123}I-labeled amines for brain studies: localization of ^{123}I-Iodophenylalkyl in rat brain. J. Nucl. Med. **21** (1980) 940–946.

[3] Hill, Th. C., P. L. Magistretti, B. L. Holman et al.: Assessment of regional cerebral blood flow (rCBF) in stroke using SPECT and N-isopropyl-(^{123}I)-p-iodoamphetamine (IMP). Stroke **15** (1984) 40–45.

[4] von Schulthess, G. K., E. Ketz, P. A. Schubiger et al.: Regional quantiative noninvasive assessment of Cerebral Perfusion and Function with N-Isopropyl-(^{123}I)p-Iodoamphetamine. J. Nucl. Med. **26** (1985) 9–16.

[5] Magistretti, P., R. Uren, D. Shomer et al.: Emission tomographic scans of cerebral blood flow using ^{123}I-iodoamphetamine in epilepsy. In: Proc. III. World Congr. Nucl. Med. & Biol. (ed.: Raynaud, C.), Pergamon Press Paris, pp. 139–143, 1982.

[6] Kreiten, K., H. J. Biersack, W. Fröscher et al.: Erste Erfahrungen mit der "Single-Photon-Emission-Computed-Tomography" (SPECT) des Gehirns bei Patienten mit Epilepsie. Act. Neurol. **12** (1985), 8–12.

[7] Todd-Pokropek, A., R. di Paola: The use of computers for image processing in nuclear medicine: IEEE Trans. Nucl. Sci. **29** (1982) 1299–1309.

[8] Shepp, L. A., B. F. Logan: Reconstructing interior head tissue from X-ray transmissions. IEEE Trans. Nucl. Sci. **21** (1974) 228–262.

[9] Bellini, S., M. Piacentini, C. Cafforio et al.: Compensation of tissue absorption in emission tomography. IEEE Trans. Acous. Speech and Sign. Proc., ASSP **27** (1979) 213–218.

[10] Budinger, Th. F.: Physical attributes of single-photon tomography. J. Nucl. Med. **21** (1980) 579–592.

[11] McKeighen, R. E., G. Muellehner, R. A. Moyer: Gamma camera collimator considerations for imaging ^{123}I. J. Nucl. Med. **15** (1974) 328–331.

[12] Waggett, D. J., B. C. Wilson: Improvement of scanner performance by subtracting of compton scattering multiple energy windows. Br. J. Rad. **51** (1978) 1004–1010.

[13] Matsui, T., A. Hirano: An Atlas of the Human Brain for Computerized Tomography. Gustav Fischer Verlag, Igaku-Shoin 1978.

[14] Phelps, M. E., J. C. Mazziota, S.-Ch. Huang: Study of Cerebral Function with Positron Computed Tomography. J. Cerebr. Blood Flow & Metabol. **2** (1982) 113–162.

[15] Kuhl, D. E., E. J. Metter, W. H. Riege et al.: Local Cerebral Glucose Utilization in elderly patients with depression, multiple infarct dementia, and Alzheimer's disease. J. Cerebr. Blood Flow & Metabol. **3** (Suppl. 1) (1983) 494–495.

[16] Goldenberg, G., I. Podreka, K. Höll et al.: rCBF changes in memorizing of verbal and nonverbal acoustic stimuli: An IMP-SPECT study. J. Cerebr. Blood Flow & Metabol. **5** (Suppl. 1) (1985) 219–220.

[17] Donley, R. F., T. M. Sundt, R. E. Anderson et al.: Blood flow measurements and the "look through" artifact in focal cerebral ischemia. Stroke **6** (1975) 121–128.

[18] Wyper, D. J., M. B. D. Cooke: Compensating for hemisphere cross-talk when measuring CBF. Acta Neurol. Scan. **56** (Suppl. 64) (1977) 470–474.

[19] Metter, E. J., W. H. Riege, D. E. Kuhl et al.: Cerebral Metabolic Relationship for Selected Brain Regions in Healthy Adults. J. Cerebr. Blood Flow & Metabol. **4** (1984) 1–7.

[20] Rapoport, S. I., B. Horowitz, R. Duara: PET scanning demonstrates that aging in man is accompanied by desynchronization of regional brain activity, without concurrent reductions in absolute cerebral metabolic rates for glucose. J. Cerebr. Blood Flow & Metabol. 5 (Suppl. 1) (1985) 119–120.

[21] Heiss, W. D., H. W. Ilsen, R. Wagner et al.: Remote functional depression of glucose metabolism in stroke and its alteration by activating drugs. In: Positron Emission Tomography of the Brain (eds.: Heiss, W. D., Phelps, M. E.), Springer Verlag, pp. 163–168, Berlin 1982.

[22] Kuhl, D. E., M. E. Phelps, A. P. Kowell: Effects of stroke on local cerebral metabolism and perfusion: mapping by emission computed tomography of 18FDG and $13NH_3$. Ann. Neurol. **8** (1980) 47–60.

[23] Lenzi, G. L., R. S. Frackowiak, T. Jones: Cerebral Oxygen Metabolism and Blood Flow in Human Cerebral Ischemic Infarction. J. Cerebr. Blood Flow & Metabol. **2** (1982) 321–335.

[24] Engel, J. Jr., W. J. Brown, D. E. Kuhl et al.: Pathological findings underlying focal temporal lobe hypometabolism in partial epilepsy. Ann. Neurol. **12** (1982) 518–528.

[25] Feindel, W., Y. Yamamoto, Ch. Thompson et al.: Positron emission tomography for cerebral blood flow measurement and detection of focal lesions in epilepsy. In: Advances in Epileptology (eds.: Canger, R., Angeleri, F., Penry, J. K.) Raven Press. pp. 73–81, New York 1980.

[26] Kuhl, D. E., J. Engel, M. E. Phelps et al.: Patterns of local cerebral metabolism and perfusion in partial epilepsy by emission computed tomography of 18F-Fluoro-deoxyglucose and 13N-Ammonia. Acta Neurol. Scan. **60** (Suppl. 72) (1979) 538–539.

[27] Yamamoto, Y. L., R. Ochs, P. Gloor et al.: Patterns of rCBF and focal energy metabolic changes in relation to electroencephalographic abnormality in inter-ictal phase of partial epilepsy. in: Cerebral Blood Flow Metabolism and Epilepsy (eds.: Baldy-Moulinier, M., Ingvar, D. H., Meldrum, B. S.), John Libbey Eurotext. pp. 51–62, London–Paris 1983.

[28] Kuhl, D. E., M. E. Phelps, C. Markham et al.: Local cerebral glucose metabolism in Huntington's disease determined by Emission Computerized Tomography of 18F-Fluorodeoxyglucose. J. Cerebr. Blood Flow & Metabol. **1** (Suppl. 1) (1981) 459–560.

[29] Metter, J., W. Riege, M. Kameyama et al.: Cerebral Metabolic Relationships for selected Brain Regions in Alzheimer's, Huntington's and Parkinson's diseases. J. Cerebr. Blood Flow & Metabol. **4** (1984) 500–506.

[30] Rougemont, D., J. C. Baron, P. Collard et al.: Local cerebral glucose utilization in treated and untreated patients with Parkinson's disease. J. Neurology, Neurosurgery & Psychatry **47** (1984) 824–830.

[31] Frackowiak, R. S. J., C. Pozilli, N. J. Legg et al.: Regional cerebral oxygen supply and utilization in dementia. A clinical and physiological study with oxygen-15 and positron tomography. Brain **104** (1981) 753–778.

[32] Baron, J. C., D. Comar, E. Zarifian et al.: Dopaminergic receptor sites in Human Brain: Positron Emission Tomography. Neurolgy **35** (1985) 16–24.

[33] Inoue, Y., H. Wagner Jr., D. Wong et al.: Atlas of Dopamine Receptor Images (PET) of the Human Brain. J. Comput. Assist. Tomogr. **9** (1985) 129–140.

[34] Frost, J. J., R. F. Danals, H. T. Ravert et al.: Imaging opiate receptors with positron emission tomography. J. Nucl. Med. **25** (1980) 73–80.

[35] Phelps, M. E., J. C. Mazziotta, D. E. Kuhl et al.: Tomographic mapping of human cerebral metabolism: visual stimulation and deprivation. Neurology **31** (1981) 517–529.

[36] Phelps, M. E., J. C. Mazziotta, J. Engel Jr.: Metabolic response of the brain to visual and auditory stimulation and deprivation. J. Cerebr. Blood Flow & Metabol. **1** (1981) 467–468.

[37] Jarritt, P. H., P. J. Ell, M. J. Meyers et al.: A new Transverse-section Brain Imager for Single-Gamma Emitters. J. Nucl. Med. **20** (1979) 319–327.

[38] Moore, S. C., H. D. Doherty, R. E. Zimmermann et al.: Improved Performance from Modifications to the Multidetector SPECT Brain Scanner. J. Nucl. Med. **25** (1984) 688–691.

[39] Lassen, N. A., E. Sveinsdottir, I. Kanno et al.: A fast single photon emission tomography system for regional cerebral blood flow studies in man. J. Comput. Assist. Tomogr. **2** (1978) 2–8.
[40] Larsson, S. A., G. Bergstrand, H. Bergstedt et al.: A special cut-off gamma camera for high resolution SPECT of the head. J. Nucl. Med. **5** (1984) 1023–1030.
[41] Esser, P. D., R. J. Mitnick, J. Arliss et al.: Angular Single Photon Emission Computed Tomography (SPECT): An improved method for cranial tomographic imaging. (paper held at SNM 30th Annual Meeting, June 1983).
[42] Madsen, M. T., Ch.-H. Park: Enhancement of SPECT Images by Fourier Filtering the Projection Image Set. J. Nucl. Med. **26** (1985) 395–402.
[43] King, M. A., R. B. Schwinger, P. W. Doherty et al.: Two-dimensional Filtering of SPECT Images using the Metz and Wiener Filters. J. Nucl. Med. **25** (1984) 1234–1240.
[44] Todd-Pokropek, A.: Image processing in nuclear medicine. IEEE Trans. Nucl. Sci. **27** (1980) 1080–1094.
[45] Engel, J. Jr.: Metabolic patterns of human epilepsy: clinical observations and possible physiological correlates. In: Cerebral Blood Flow Metabolism and Epilepsy (eds.: Baldy-Moulinier, M., Ingvar, D. H., Meldrum, B. S.). John Libbey Eurotext. pp. 6–18, London–Paris, 1983.
[46] Kuhl, D. E., E. L. Wu, T. H. Lin et al.: Mapping local cerebral blood flow by means of emission computed tomography of N-Isopropyl-p(^{123}I)-Iodoamphetamine (IMP). J. Cerebr. Blood Flow & Metabol. **1** (Suppl. 1) (1981) 25–26.
[47] Kuhl, D. E., J. R. Barrio, S. Ch. Huang et al.: Quantifying local cerebral blood flow by N-Isopropyl-p(^{123}I)-Iodoamphetamine (IMP) tomography. J. Nucl. Med. **23** (1982) 196–203.
[48] Raynaud, C., G. Rancurel, Y. Samson et al.: Measurement of oxygen metabolism, ^{123}I-IMP distribution and rCBF-Xe in patients with ischemic vascular disease. J. Nucl. Med. **25** (1984) 8.
[49] Büll, U., C. M. Kirsch, V. Olteanu-Nerbe et al.: Results of ^{123}I-Amphetamine single photon emission CT (SPECT) as compared to ^{133}Xenon dynamic SPECT. In: ^{123}I-Amphetamine (Perfusamine TM) (eds.: von Schulthess, G. K., Bekier, A., Schubiger, P. A.) Editiones “Roche”. pp. 91–105, Basle 1983.
[50] Podreka, I., K. Höll, P. Dal Bianco et al.: Klinische und technische Aspekte der SPECT-Hirnscintigraphie mit ^{123}J-N-Isopropyl-Amphetamin. NucCompact **6** (1984) 305–314.
[51] Hedde, J. P., W. Fiegler, R. Schneider et al.: Dynamische SPECT zur Messung der cerebralen ^{123}J-Amphetamin-Kinetik. NucCompact **6** (1984) 330–226.
[52] Lassen, N. A., L. Henriksen, O. Paulson: Regional Cerebral Blood Flow in stroke by ^{133}Xenon inhalation and Emission Tomography. Stroke **12** (1981) 284–288.
[53] Hoffman, E. J., S. Ch. Huang, M. E. Phelps: Quantitation in positron emission computed tomography: 1. Effect of object size. J. Comput. Assist. Tomogr. **3** (1979) 299–308.
[54] Mazziotta, J. C., M. E. Phelps, D. Plummer et al.: Quantitation in positron emission computed tomography: 5. Physical-anatomical effects. J. Comput. Assist. Tomogr. **5** (1981) 734–743.

Regional iodoamphetamine (^{123}I-IMP) Uptake (SPECT) and Regional Cerebral Blood Flow (^{133}Xe-DSPECT)

U. Buell, W. Krappel, P. Schmiedek, K. Einhäupl

Regional cerebral blood flow (rCBF) may be measured employing inhalation of ^{133}Xe-gas either by probes or by a specially designed DSPECT machine [1, 6]. Results are rCBF values in ml/100 g/min.
Assumptions, inherent in the calculations, are well known [9]. However, in a large series of patients with cerebrovascular disease (CVD), we and others found excellent correlation of rCBF to clinical presentation, angiographic findings or results of transmission CT [1, 6].

^{123}I-amphetamine (IMP), as a lipophilic tracer, is distributed in correlation to rCBF beyond the blood-brain-barrier [3, 4, 8] and was found to keep this correlative distribution unchanged for more than one hour [4]. However, we and other groups experienced visually a change in distribution with increasing time after injection [2, 7].

The present study in patients with CVD is aimed at comparing interhemispherical ratios of rCBF (derived from ^{133}Xe-DSPECT, right-to-left or diseased-to-nondiseased) to ratios from corresponding IMP slices, in correlation to time after injection of IMP, and to different sizes of regions of interest used for slice evaluation. Thus, we sought to identify by ratios differences or congruence of Xenon and IMP.

Moreover, regional IMP uptake (counts/mCi/pixel) was determined in selected regions (normal or diseased) at different periods of time after injection. By this design, experience could be gained on regional behaviour of IMP depending on the state of brain tissue, as documented by TCT and clinical presentation.

Patients and methods

This study includes 20 patients with cerebrovascular disease (19 male, 1 female), who had strictly unilateral changes in cranial vasculature (stenosis or occlusion of the ICA, main cerebral arteries or both). Thus, patients were separated by invasive cranial angiography.

Within one week the following examinations were done:
- Clinical examination
- Transmission CT
- Cranial angiography
- ^{133}Xe DSPECT
- IMP-DSPECT

^{133}Xe-DSPECT

Dynamic SPECT was done with a Tomomatic 64 (Medimatic, Copenhagen, Denmark) which is described in detail elsewhere [6]. In short, after inhalation of ^{133}Xe-gas from a special system (370 MBq/1 l), a four detector array system rotates around the patient's head with 6 rpm. After one minute inhalation and three minutes exhalation, by employing the Kanno-Lassen algorithm [5], the results are displayed as flow maps in transaxial slices (three slices of 20 mm thickness by collimation) in a 32 × 32 matrix. The colour coded flow maps represent ml/100 g/min.

IMP-SPECT

A dual head Rota-camera (Siemens-Gammasonics) was used after i.v. injection of 175 MBq ^{123}I-IMP (p, 5n). One total rotation took only 14 min., since either head rotates 180° (in step and shoot, delivering 32 angle projections each). This procedure was performed three times after injection, 13–27 min., 33–47 min., and 5,5 hrs. p.i.. Reconstruction was done employing a Delta-system (CDA, Hamburg), establishing slices of IMP distribution of three pixels thickness (20 mm) on a 64 × 64 matrix.

Evaluation

Evaluation of ^{133}Xe-DSPECT and IMP-SPECT was done visually and by computer programs on identical Xenon and IMP slices, which were selected (two slices per patient) by anatomical landmarks. For comparison, the same region of interest program (fig. 1a) was employed, framing two half slices or six regions per half slice. In Xenon or IMP, right-to-left and diseased-to-nondiseased interhemispherical ratios were obtained within two representatives slices:
A) from half slices (two ratios per patient) and
B) from areas (six ratios per slice, 12 ratios per patient).

Moreover, IMP-slices were evaluated by an additional computer program, designed to separate grey matter und basal ganglia (fig. 1b). Thus, IMP counts were measured per area, decay corrected, and calibrated to injected activity (measured in a dose calibrator) and to one minute (fig. 1b). The result was counts/min/pixel/mCi. For inter-IMP comparison, data determined 33–47 min. p.i. were used as the reference

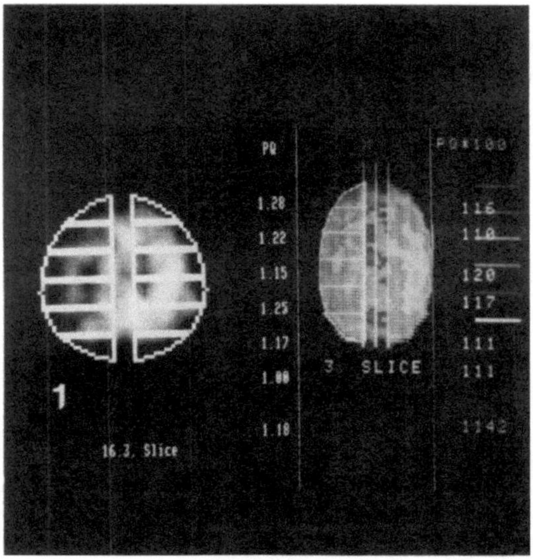

a

Fig. 1 31-year old patient, occluded left ICA and history of TIA. Identical slices (a) from ^{123}I-IMP (left, time 1 = 13–27 min. p.i.) and ^{133}Xe-DSPECT (right). ROIs, derived from routine Xe-DSPECT revealed PQ (= right-to-left-ratios) for Xe-*areas* (1.28–1.00) and IMP-areas (1.16–1.11) or Xe-*half slices* (bottom: 1.18) and IMP-half slices (1.142) (a). Evaluation of identical IMP-slices with specially designed IMP-ROI (b) at examination times 1 to 3 (13–27 min., 33–47 min. and 5.5. hrs p.i.) displayed increasing (normalized and decay corrected) countrates in diseased areas of the left hemisphere or increasing (1 to 2) and thereafter decreasing (2 to 3) counts in normal brain (right hemisphere), corresponding to visual findings of "filling in" (c, arrows). Right-to-left ratios (PQ) changed (b) from 1 to 3. *Continued: see pages 130, 131.*

(= 100%) for uptake values from 13–27 min. or 5,5 hrs. p.i. (fig. 2). To separate various stages of disease, the difference to the contralateral density was used. To exclude ratios from not involved hemispherical regions from the correlation, differences of less than 11% (half-slice) or 14% (areas) at IMP 1 (13–27 min. p.i.) were excluded. In inter-IMP comparison, defects were additionally weighted by an arbitrary 20% threshold. For arithmetic comparison, all data were displayed as 1.00 minus diseased-to-nondiseased countrates. For graphic comparison (fig. 3) the right-to-left ratio were used. In addition, the size of defects in Xenon-DSPECT or IMP-SPECT were compared to the size of low density areas in TCT-slices.

Results

Xenon vs IMP

Comparative results of half slice-ratios for all patients or patients with an interhemispherical difference of > 0.11 (11%) at IMP_1 are given in tables 1 or 2. In either groups IMP_1 differences were very close to Xenon differences. However, with increasing time after injection of IMP, IMP values became smaller. Correlation

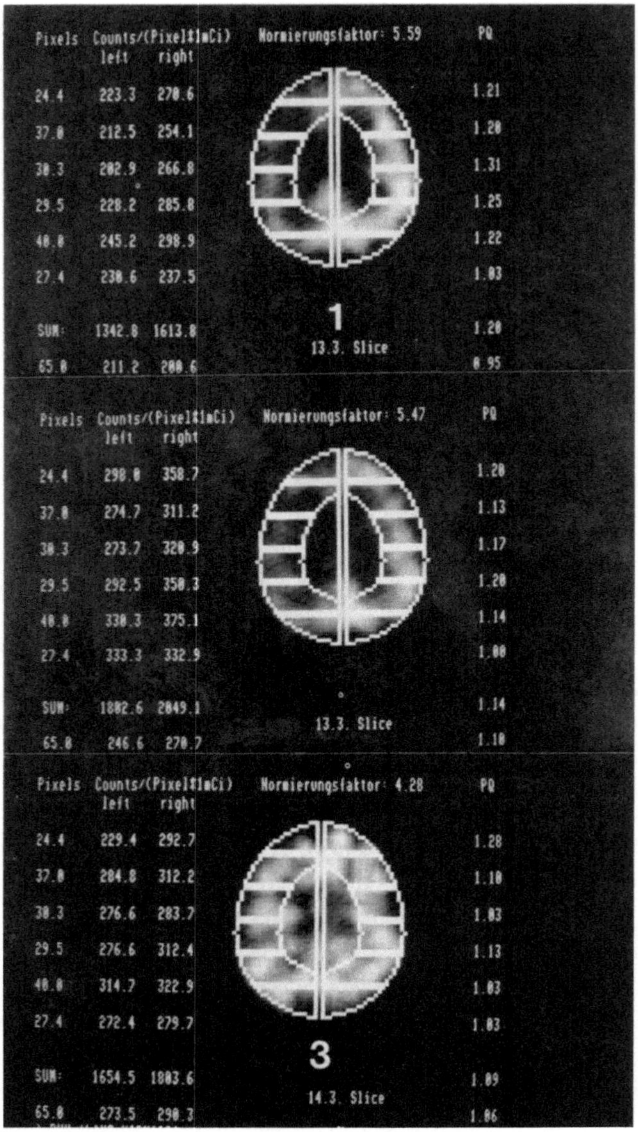

b

Fig. 1 *(Continued)*

coefficient r, therefore, decreased from 0.84 to 0.14 or from 0.82 to 0.35. In the group of interhemispherical differences, exceeding a threshold of 0.11 (tab. 2), significant differences of IMP to Xenon were already found for IMP_2 (time 2 = 33–47 min.).

A graphic display corresponding to table 1 is given in fig. 3. for right-to-left-ratios. The deviation from the line of identity increases with time elapsed, from time 1 (13–27 min.) to 3 (5.5 hrs. p.i.).

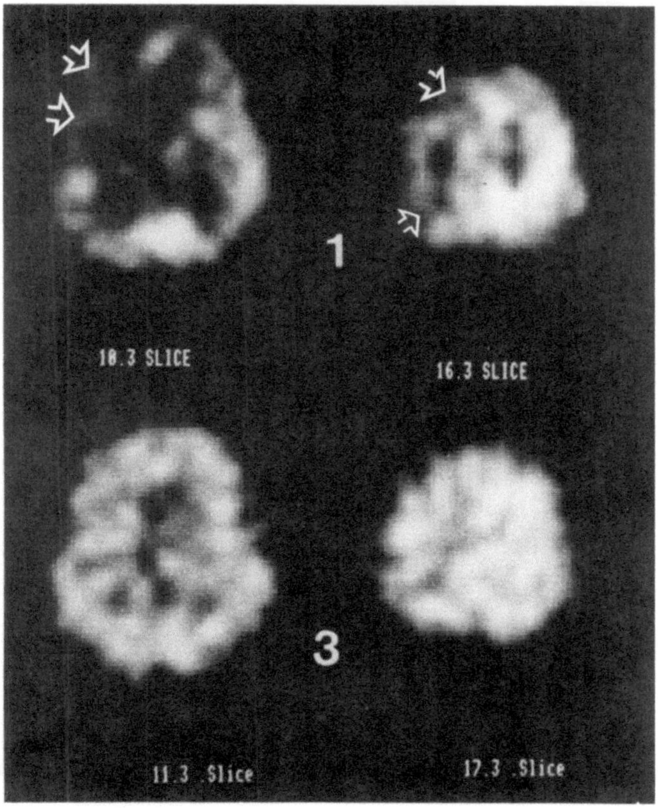

c

Fig. 1 *(Continued)*

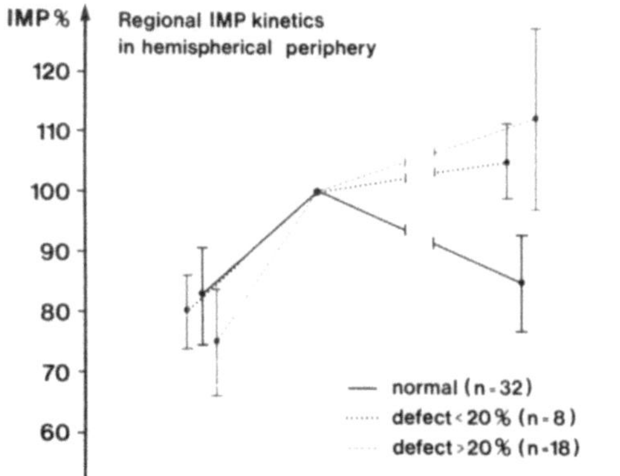

Fig. 2 Regional IMP kinetics in hemispherical areas, normalized to the countrates at 33–47 min. (40) p.i. Mind increase in defected areas ("filling in") vs. decrease in normal areas. Larger defects (> 20% difference to contralateral areas) increased more than smaller defects (< 20%).

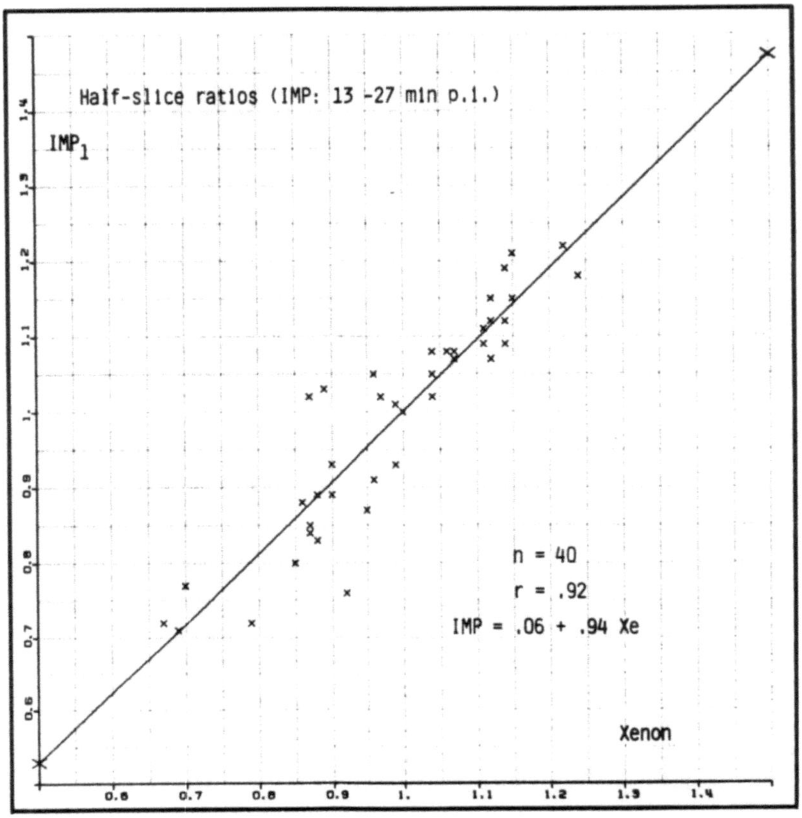

a

Fig. 3 Correlation of IMP vs. Xenon half slice ratios (right-to-left) at time 1 (a), 2 (b) and 3 (c). Mind that inclusion of normal ratios (0.90–1.10) yields higher correlation coefficients at time 2 (b, r = 0.92) than exclusion (tab. 2). However, intercept decreases from 1 to 3.
Cotinued: see pages 133, 134

If the areal ratios were compared (fig. 1a, tab. 3) and an threshold for interhemispherical differences was set at 0.14 (14%), such differences obtained from low flow areas where considerably greater than from half-slices (tab. 2). The IMP-values descreased with time elapsed from 1 to 3.

Regional IMP kinetics in various brain areas

The results are given in table 4. In normal brain areas, IMP uptake (related to IMP_2) increased from 1 to 2 and decreased from 2 to 3. In defected areas (tab. 5), the increase from 1 to 2 was greater (25% in large defects) than in normal periphery (17,5%). In ganglia, similar results were found. From 2 to 3, normal hemispherical uptake decreased by 15.2%. However, in defects, a further increase was measured (5–12%). The same effect occurred in ganglia. These results are displayed graphically in fig. 2.

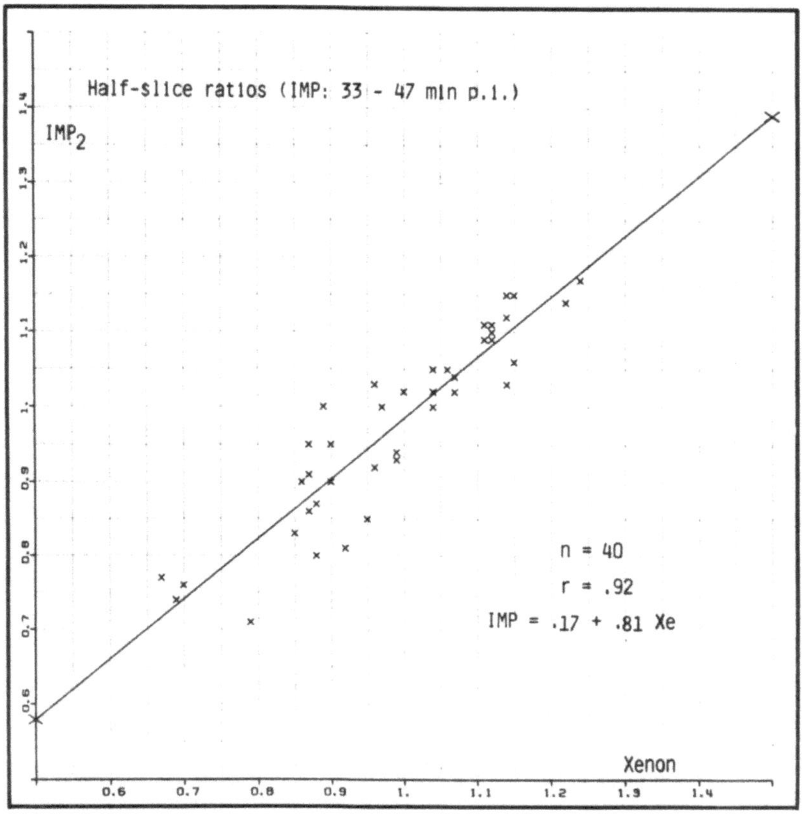

b

Fig. 3 *(Continued)*

Table 1 Comparison of half-slice ratios: ^{133}Xe vs $IMP_{1,2,3}$§ (all patients)

	n	mean ± SD	r
Xe	40	.111 ± .08	–
IMP_1	40	.118 ± .08	.82
IMP_2	40	.101 ± .07	.78
IMP_3	40	.055 ± .05	.35

§ displayed as 1.00 minus diseased/normal 1,2,3 = 13–27 min, 33–47 min, 5,5 hrs p. i.
Xe vs 1:p<.15; vs 2:p<.10; vs 3:p<.005

Table 2 Comparison of half-slice ratios: ^{133}Xe vs $IMP_{1,2,3}$ (threshold: .110)§

	n	mean ± SD	r
Xe	18	.173 ± .07	–
IMP_1	18	.175 ± .06	.84
IMP_2	18	.148 ± .07	.72
IMP_3	18	.076 ± .05	.14

§ at IMP_1, as a result of 1.00 minus diseased/normal. 1–3: time p. i.
Xe vs 1:p<.15; vs 2:p<.025; vs 3:p<.01

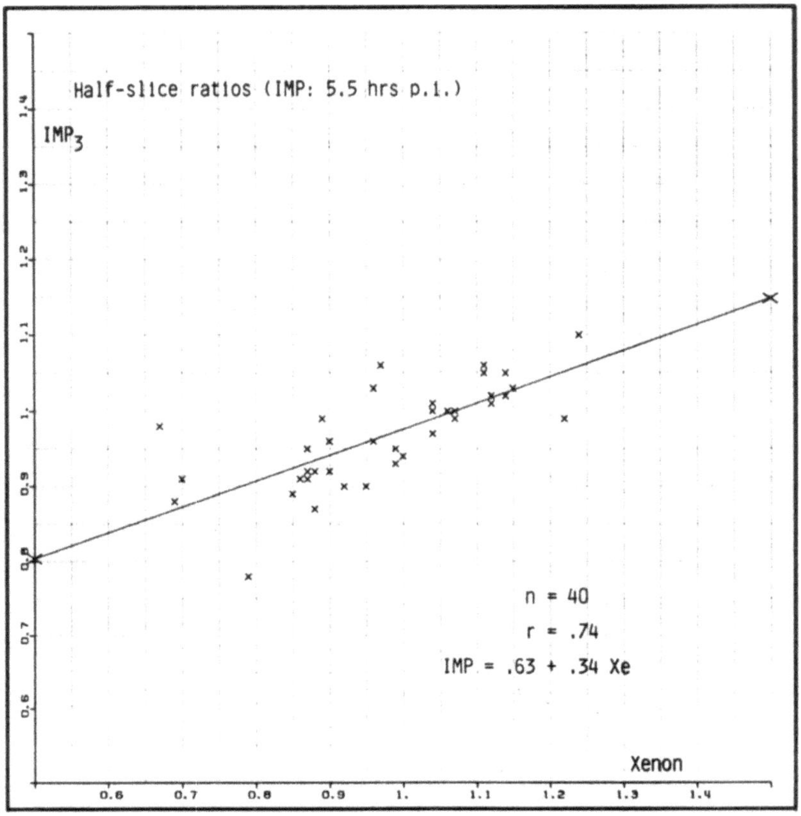

c

Fig. 3 *(Continued)*

Table 3 Comparison of areal ratios: ^{133}Xe vs $IMP_{1,2,3}$ (threshold: .140)[§]

	n	mean ± SD	r
Xe	21	.262 ± .08	–
IMP_1	21	.270 ± .07	.61
IMP_2	21	.233 ± .07	.33
IMP_3	21	.106 ± .07	.03

§ at IMP_1, as a result of 1.00 minus diseased/normal. 1–3: time p. i.
Xe vs 1:$p<.5$; vs 2:$p<.15$; vs 3:$p<.001$

Table 4 Regional IMP kinetics in various normal brain areas

Area	n	IMP_1/IMP_2	IMP_3/IMP_2
hemispherical periphery	32	.825 ± .08	.848 ± .08
frontal periphery	30	.820 ± .09	.850 ± .09
occipital periphery	30	.830 ± .08	.840 ± .09
basal ganglia	15	.815 ± .08	.910 ± .09

meas. performed at min 13–27 (IMP_1), 33–47 ($_2$) and hrs 5.5 ($_3$) after inj. double-elliptic ROI design

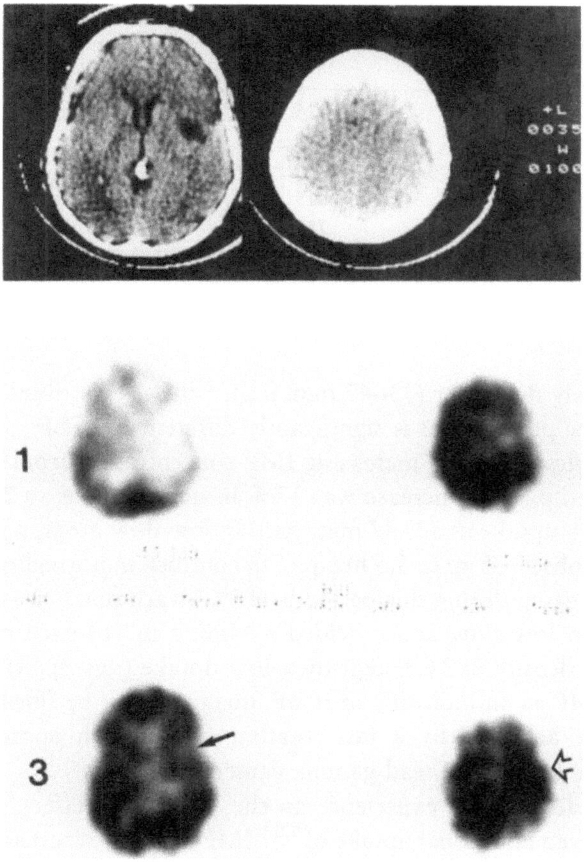

a

b

Fig. 4 51-year old patient, stenosis of left ICA; history of PRIND. TCT (a) revealed a low density defect in the right hemisphere, temporo-parietal region. No defect in the parietal areas. IMP (b) at 13–27 min. (1) p.i. showed low perfusion throughout the whole temporal and parts of the parietal (right hemisphere. "Filling in" occurred at 5.5 hrs (3), except defected area (solid arrow). In parietal regions of the right hemisphere, maximum uptake is displayed at 3 (contour arrow).

At 1 (13–27 min. p.i.), a visual comparison of the size of low uptake areas in IMP to the size of low density areas in TCT revealed in every singly case a more extended low uptake area (fig. 4). However, at 3 (5.5 hrs. p.i.), such areas in IMP slices shrunk dramatically by size. This effect was not observed if density values (TCT) were close or identical with CSF (fig. 4). In some cases, low uptake areas at 1 showed maximal counts at 3 (fig. 4).

Conclusions

1. If rCBF ratios from ^{133}Xe-DSPECT were used as a "gold standard", ^{123}I-IMP uptake was well correlated to rCBF in the early phase of the distribution (13–27 min.).

Table 5 Regional IMP kinetics in hemispherical periphery and ganglia

Area	n	IMP_1/IMP_2	IMP_3/IMP_2
normal	32	.825 ± .08	.848 ± .08
defect<20%[a]	8	.800 ± .06	1.050 ± .09
defect>20%[b]	18	.750 ± .09	1.120 ± .15
normal ganglia	15	.815 ± .08	.910 ± .09
defect. ganglia[c]	9	.780 ± .05	1.120 ± .12

meas. performed at min 13–27 (IMP_1), 33–47 ($_2$) and hrs 5.5 ($_3$) after inj. double-elliptic (ROI) design mean "defect" differences-to-normal (a, b, c): 18% (a), 29% (b) or 18% (c).

2. Commencing immediately thereafter (33–47 min. p.i.), ^{123}I-IMP distribution and uptake changes to a new pattern that is significantly different to rCBF.
3. Regional ^{123}I-IMP kinetics led to an increasing IMP-concentration from 13–27 min. i.p. to 33–47 min. i.p.. This increase was 17% in normal areas vs 25% in low flow areas (100% = uptake at 33–47 min. p.i.). In low flow areas, a further increase of 5–12% was observed up to 5.5 hrs. p.i.. In contrast, in normal regions, IMP-concentration decreased during this period by 15% (wash out > wash in?).
4. This increase of IMP in low flow areas yielded a "filling in" of such defects. However, areas of CSF density in TCT kept their low uptake (figs. 1c, 4).
5. Thus, to employ ^{123}I-IMP as an indicator of rCBF, imaging must be finished 30 min. p.i.. This may be achieved by a fast rotating system with appropriate resolution, preferrably by a double-head gamma camera.
6. Further studies are needed to gain experience on the "filling in" effect. It may reflect either a very delayed additional uptake of ^{123}I-IMP in low flow areas (wash in > wash out) or an additional uptake of IMP metabolites in low flow but still viable areas.

References

[1] Buell, U., E. A. Moser, P. Schmiedek et al.: Dynamic SPECT with ^{133}Xe: regional cerebral Blood flow in patients with unilateral cerebrovascular Disease: concise communication. J. Nucl. Med. **25** (1984) 441–446.

[2] Buell, U., P. Schmiedek, C. M. Kirsch et al.: Interhemispherical ratios of perfusion in ^{123}I-amphetamine SPECT and ^{133}Xe dynamic SPECT. A comparative study in patients with cerebrovascular disease (CVD). In: Nuclear Medicine in Research and Practice (eds.: H. A. E. Schmidt, D. E. Vauramo), F. K. Schattauer, Stuttgart–New York, 1984, p. 435.

[3] Ell, P. J., I. Cullum, M. Donaghy et al.: Cerebral blood flow studies with ^{123}Jodine-labelled Amines. Lancet. June 18 (1983) 1348.

[4] Hill, T. C., P. L. Magistretti, L. Holman et al.: Assessment of regional cerebral blood flow (rCBF) in stroke using SPECT and N-isopropyl-(^{123}I)-p-iodoamphetamine (IMP). Stroke **15** (1984) 40–45.

[5] Kanno, I., N. A. Lassen: Two methods for calculating regional cerebral blood flow from emission computed tomography of inert gas concentrations. J. Comp. Ass. Tomogr. **3** (1979) 71–76.

[6] Lassen, N. A., L. Henriksen, O. Paulson: Regional cerebral blood flow in stroke by ^{133}Xenon inhalation and emission tomography. Stroke **12** (1981) 284–288.

[7] Raynaud, C., G. Rancurel, Y. Samson et al.: Measurement of oxygen metabolism, ^{123}I-IMP distribution and rCBF-Xe in patients with ischemic vascular disease. (Abstr.). J. nucl. Med. **25** (1984) P8.

[8] Schulthess, v. G. K., E. Ketz, P. A. Schubiger et al.: Regional quantitative noninvasive assessment of cerebral perfusion and function with N-Isopropyl-(^{123}I)p-Iodoamphetamine. J. nucl. Med. **26** (1985) 9–16.

[9] Stokely, E. M., E. Sveinsdottir, N. A. Lassen et al.: A single photon dynamic computer assisted tomograph (DCAT) for imaging brain function in multiple cross sections. J. Comp. Ass. Tomogr. **4** (1980) 230--240.

Regional Quantification of SPECT-Studies of the Brain with N-Isopropyl-[^{123}I]p-Iodo-Amphetamine (IMP)

G. K. von Schulthess, A. Meili, B. Weder, A. Bekier

Abstract

Sixteen SPECT-studies were performed on fifteen normal volunteers and quantitatively analyzed using a fixed set of seven paired regions of interest, matching cerebral perfusion territories. The regions corresponded to territories supplied by the anterior, middle (3 regions) and posterior cerebral arteries, the basal ganglia and the cerebellar hemispheres. Right to left ratios were found to be close to 1 with standard deviations of <2%. The usefulness of the quantification scheme implemented in this paper and elsewhere [1] is discussed and illustrated with the studies of four patients, two suffering from cerebrovascular disease, one from a cerebellar abscess and one from epilepsy, respectively.

Introduction

N-isopropyl-[^{123}I]p-iodoamphetamine (IMP) scanning has been in use in Europe for more than two years, and several reports on its clinical usefulness have appeared in the literature [1–6]. As reduced tissue perfusion results in decreased cerebral IMP uptake [1, 2], patients with cerebrovascular disease have been primarily examined with this substance. However, IMP-uptake requires not only adequate perfusion, but also intact function of brain tissue; IMP has thus been termed a perfusion/function marker [1]. As a result, tumors and other mass lesions do not show IMP-uptake [7]. On the other hand, patients with cerebral hyperactivity, such as seen during an epileptic attack show increased IMP-uptake, and some authors have suggested that IMP-studies may be useful in the evaluation of such patients [8].

Based on our experience with by now over 170 SPECT (*S*ingle *P*hoton *E*mission *C*omputed *T*omography) studies on patients, we have implemented a regional quantification scheme, presented elsewhere [1], which uses symmetrical regions of interest (ROI), corresponding to vascular perfusion territories. Quantification was found to be useful in preventing false positive and false negative diagnoses, which may result from simple qualitative evaluation of SPECT scans [1]. The vascular territories quantified by the symmetrical paired regions were the territories of the anterior, middle and posterior cerebral arteries, and the basal ganglia. The purpose of this presentation is to extend this quantitative analysis to the cerebellum, which has been found to exhibit contralateral decreased functional activity in patients with hemispheric insults [9], and to present three cases to illustrate when such quantitative analysis appears particularly useful.

Patients and methods

15 normals underwent 16 IMP SPECT-studies according to a protocol described elsewhere [1]. The same protocol was used for all patients. Data were acquired with the patients orbito-meatal plane perpendicular to the rotation axis of the SPECT camera. A single head PICKER Dyna-scan camera equipped with a Micro-Z digital homogeneity correction was used for imaging. 60 projections over a full 360° camera rotation were acquired, taking a total of 25 to 35 min (20 or 30 sec per projection), and yielding 30 000 to 50 000 counts per projection or a total of $1.8–3.0 \times 10^6$ counts per study. The distance of the camera surface to the axis of rotation was 20 to 25 cm depending on the patient.

Data were stored and analyzed in a KETRONIC Medax-N desktop computer. The raw data were reconstructed without attenuation correction by the backprojection method using a Shepp-Logan filter [10]. Slice thickness was two pixels corresponding to 1.2 cm. Care was taken to position the top six slices on the anterior projection such that the lowest slice contained information from the base of the brain. This was rechecked in the reconstructed images by noting activity in the basal ganglia on slices 5 and 6. For quantitative analysis the slices were added in pairs and

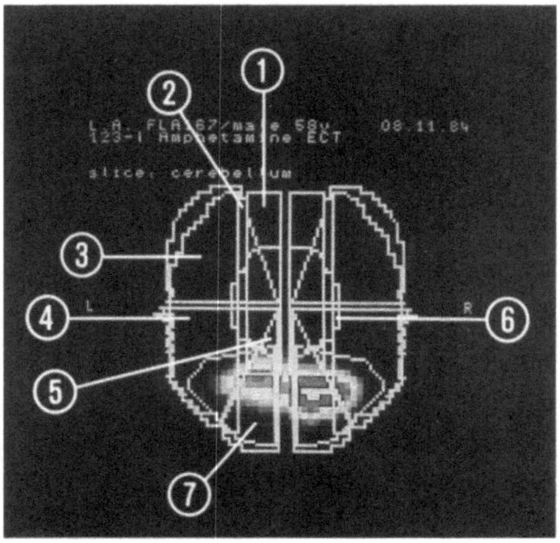

Fig. 1 IMP-SPECT of normal volunteer of the level of the cerebellum. Superimposed are 7 pairs of symmetrical regions of interest covering various perfusion territories. For the slice presented here only the values of the cerebellar regions are obtained. Also in other slices only the pixel counts in the appropriate regions are obtained, although the computer always yield the pixel count for all regions.

the resulting images smoothed once, such that there were three 2.4 cm slices above the skull base and one to two slices through the cerebellum. 7 pairs of symmetrical ROI's were used. They encompassed the perfusion territories of (1) the anterior cerebral arteries, (2) the superior, (3) anterior and (4) posterior parts of the middle cerebral arteries, (5) the posterior cerebral arteries, (6) the deep perforator arteries and (7) the arteries supplying the cerebellar hemispheres. (1) and (2) were in the top slice, (3) to (5) in the middle slice, (6) in the slice at the skull base and (7) in one of the cerebellar slices. The ROI's were drawn with a light pen on the computer screen on one study and saved in a file for repeated use, because it was felt that the variations in cerebral anatomy were small compared to the errors which could have been introduced by redrawing the regions for each patient. In addition, recalling the regions rather than redrawing them resulted in considerable savings of analysis time. The shape of the ROI's were defined based on recently published anatomical work [11]. The reconstructed SPECT images were brought to registration with the ROI's by shifting them on the computer screen. Figure 1 shows all 14 ROI's on an image at the level of the cerebellum.

Results

The results obtained by quantitatively analyzing the 16 normal studies are summarized in table 1. Ratios are given for the right to left sided pixel count for each symmetrical pair of regions, i.e. the territory of the anterior cerebral artery, three subterritories of the middle cerebral artery, the territory of the posterior cerebral artery, the basal ganglia and the cerebellum. It is important to note, that these ratios are very close to 1 with standard deviations between 1.5 and 2%. All ratios are slightly above 1, but except for region (3), the difference for 1 is well within a standard deviation.

Table 1 Normal right/left ratios of IMP distribution (mean and standard deviation)

Region of Interest		mean R/L-ratio	standard deviation
anterior cerebral artery	(1)	1.004	0.012
middle cerebral artery			
-superior territory	(2)	1.006	0.018
-anterior territory	(3)	1.021	0.016
-posterior territory	(4)	1.004	0.014
posterior cerebral artery	(5)	0.998	0.018
basal ganglia	(6)	1.011	0.013
cerebellum	(7)	1.002	0.015
age		44	18

Case studies

Case 1

51 year old caucasian male who presented with a history of transient ischemic attacks was admitted to the hospital with a prolonged ischemic event. A work-up including angiography showed occlusion of the left internal carotid artery. Quantification of the right/left ratios for regions (1)–(7) is given in table 2 (Case 1a). There is a very abnormal R/L ratio for region (3), and less so for region (2) correctly localizing the deficit on the left. The slice through a mid-level of the cerebral hemisphere is shown in fig. 2a, and also demonstrates the deficit.

The patient subsequently underwent an extracranial-intracranial bypass operation and his intermittent right sided symptomatology improved. A repeat IMP-study yielded the results given under the heading case 1b in table 2, the corresponding image being shown in fig. 2b. Although the quantitative analysis shows a significant decrease in the R/L ratio in territory (3) from 1.116 to 1.004, it is much more difficult to appreciate this change by only inspecting the images. Region (2) shows now normal values, whereas region (1) becomes slightly subnormal.

a 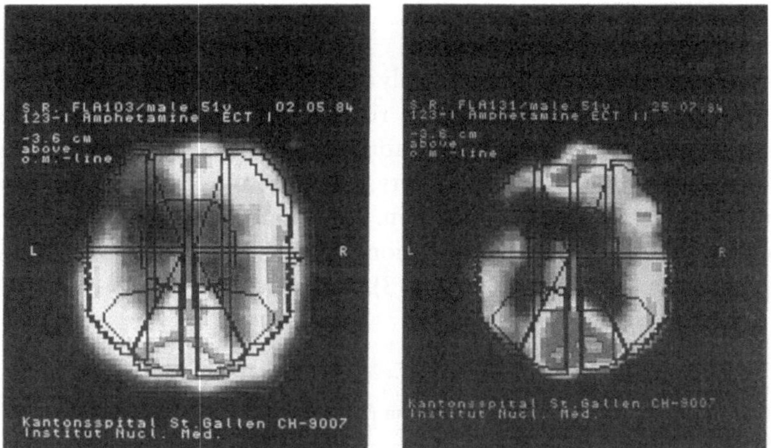 b

Fig. 2 Slices centered at 3.6 cm above the orbito-meatal line through lateral ventricles and centrum semiovale of a patient with cerebral ischemia a) pre- and b) post extracranial-intracranial bypass operation. Note anterior left sided IMP deficit on both scans.

Case 2

A 58 year old caucasian male presented with left hemisyndrome. An IMP SPECT demonstrated a perfusion deficit in the right hemisphere (fig. 3). Quantitative analysis showed marked decrease in the R/L ratio, most prominently in the MCA territory, consistent with the stroke in this region. Note that of all R/L ratios only the cerebellar one favors the right, a phenomenon known as cerebellar diaschisis [9].

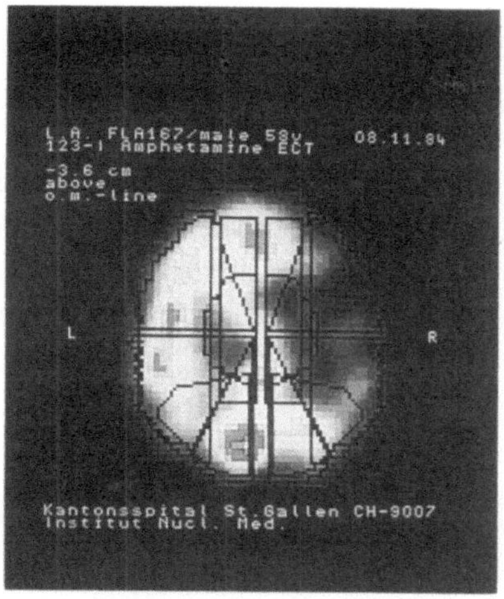

Fig. 3 Patient with established insult to the right hemisphere. Note, how the deficit in IMP is limited to the pie-piece shaped regions of the MCA territory on the right.

Case 3

51 year old caucasian female presenting with status post drainage of a right cerebellar abscess (fig. 4a). The deficit is clearly seen in fig. 4a and the highly pathological cerebellar R/L ratio is noted in table 2. Even though fig. 4b suggests an asymmetry favoring the right, this interpretation is not supported by quantitative analysis.

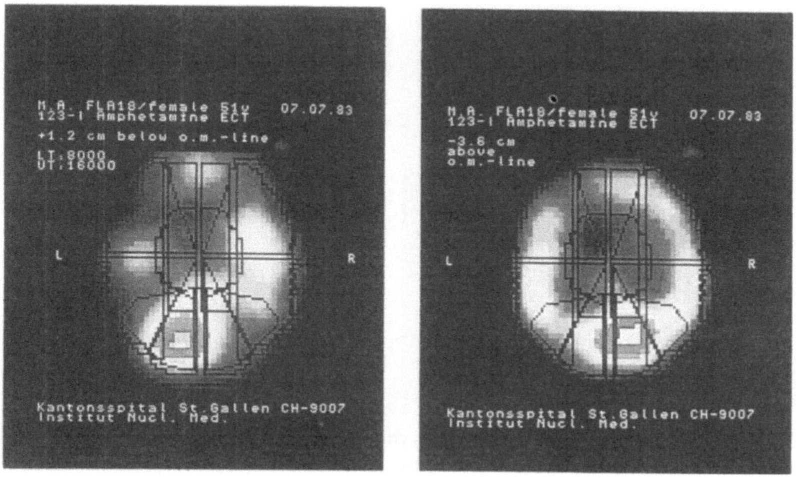

a b

Fig. 4 Patient status post drainage of a right cerebellar abscess, a) showing IMP deficit in that area. b) In the section 3.6 cm above the orbito-meatal line a slight left anterior perfusion deficit is noted whose presence is not confirmed by quantitative right/left comparison.

Case 4

5½ year old male who suffered from tonic clonic seizures predominantly affecting his left shoulder. An ictal IMP-study revealed increased uptake in the right motor cortex consistent with the clinical picture. Figure 5a is an axial section showing the right sided hot spot. Two sagittal images (figs. 5b and c) to the right of the midline delineate the hyperactive area to better advantage and clearly localize the increased cerebral perfusion/function in the motor area of the right cortex of this patient. Quantitative analysis of the R/L ratios is given in table 2 and confirms the predominance of right cerebral activity.

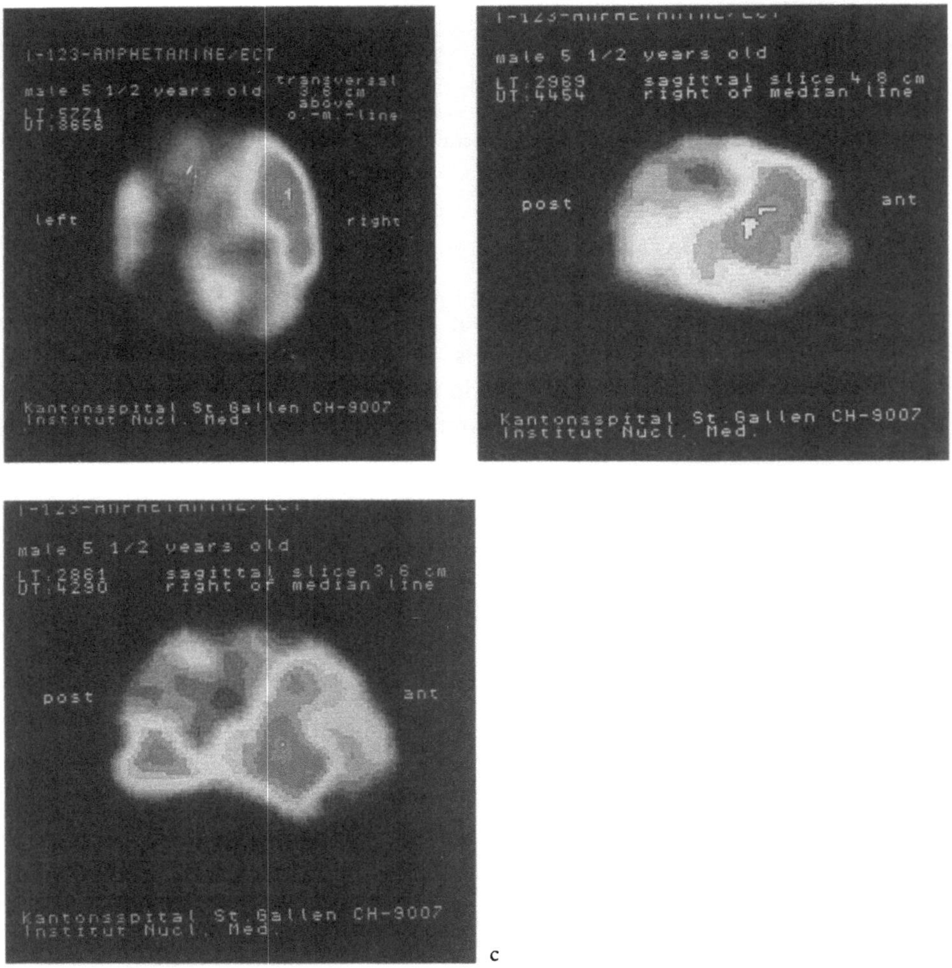

a b c

Fig. 5 5½ year old patient with epilepsia partialis continua. No regions are superimposed as this is not a cerebrovascular patient. a) There is a region of increased right sided IMP-uptake in the fronto-parietal area. Localization of this region is made to better advantage on two sagittal scans b) and c) lateral to the midline, falling clearly in the region of the motor cortex, and corresponding to the epileptic focus.

Table 2 Right/left ratios in some patients

Region of Interest		Case 1a	Case 1b	Case 2	Case 3	Case 4
anterior cerebral artery	(1)	0.985	0.952	0.968	1.019	1.014
middle cerebral artery						
-superior territory	(2)	1.050	1.015	0.913	1.016	0.977
-anterior territory	(3)	1.116	1.044	0.851	1.028	1.026
-posterior territory	(4)	0.988	1.010	0.918	1.010	1.036
posterior cerebral artery	(5)	1.013	0.978	0.985	1.007	1.051
basal ganglia	(6)	0.979	1.004	0.964	1.030	1.036
cerebellum	(7)	1.006	1.019	1.033	0.088	1.066
age/sex		51/M	51/M	58/M	51/F	51/2/M

Discussion

The data presented here confirm and extend the experience previously gained with this method [1]. First, a very narrow deviation from a R/L ratio of 1 is found in normals. This emphasizes that there is very little cerebral asymmetry, as detected with IMP. Based on the results presented here, the same appears true for the cerebellum. Similar results are found using Positron Emission Computed Tomography [12].

The advantages of our quantitative assessment of right/left asymmetry are illustrated with the cases presented here.

1. When serial studies are performed on one patient, calculation and comparison of the R/L ratios permits one to quantitatively assess disease progress or improvement. This is illustrated in case 1, where IMP-SPECT was used to evaluate the result of an extracranial-intracranial bypass operation. The study presented here suggested that the cerebral perfusion/function state of this patient had improved considerably. This was confirmed be the patients clinical presentation. Renewed angiographic evaluation showed patency of the anastomosis. It has been found previously that IMP distribution closely correlates with the clinical presentation [1].

2. Due to the somewhat arbitrary setting of the color scale on IMP-studies, a visual assessment of IMP uptake can be misleading. The normalization of the R/L ratios in case 1 mainly in the anterior MCA territory (3) is not evident from a comparison of the images in figs. 2a and 2b. Even though on inspection there is asymmetry in fig. 4 not only in the cerebellum but also in the hemispheres, this impression is not confirmed by quantitative analysis. A mismatch between the visual impression and quantitative result cautions us to call a study positive or negative, thus helping to prevent primarily false positive diagnoses which, due to the inhomogeneous cerebral IMP uptake even in normals, are inevitable.

3. Case 2 illustrates a frequent finding in patients with cerebral insults i.e. that the cerebellar hemisphere contralateral to the affected cerebral hemisphere shows decreased IMP uptake. This phenomenon termed cerebellar diaschisis, has been also observed in PET-studies [9] and seems to be the result of decreased cerebellar input from the diseased hemisphere through the crossed cortico-ponto-cerebellar nerve tract. Case 3 suggests visually, that there also exists something like a "reverse diaschisis" resulting in contralateral cerebral hypofunction from an insult to the cerebellum, in this case a cerebellar abscess. However, quantitative analysis puts in doubt such a conclusion and in addition, an anatomical basis for such a correlation is lacking (Heiss WD, contribution to the discussion of this case at the IMP-workshop in Bonn).

4. The regional quantitative analyses proposed here and elsewhere [1] was specifically designed for diagnosing cerebrovascular disease, for which IMP SPECT holds the greatest potential. Therefore, perfusion territory matched regional quantitative analysis is less suitable for patients with epileptic disease such as case 4. However, the R/L ratios given for this case in table 2 demonstrate that the changes in IMP uptake which can be expected in epileptic patients in the ictal state are more subtle than in ischemic disease. Furthermore, epileptic foci show an area of increased rather than decreased IMP uptake.

A major drawback of the usefulness of the IMP SPECT studies presented here is their limited spatial resolution (2.0–2.5 cm), which only permits artefact free assessment of relatively large pathological findings. Therefore, the perfusion territories delineated by our regions of interest where chosen to be large, and utilization of these regions for all patients appears possible despite normal anatomical variations. With an improvement of spatial resolution to the 1.0–1.5 cm range, which appears possible with present-day SPECT-systems (see contribution of Podreka et al.) and new Gamma-camera developments (which permit rotations closer to the patients head by either modification of the Gamma-camera head or the use of a slant-hole collimator) considerable gains in the diagnostic potential of IMP-SPECT studies are to be expected. The relatively crude design of our regions of interest may then become inappropriate. Anatomic ROI definition program such as the one implemented by Buell and coworkers also described in this book, may thus have to be used.

Acknowledgment

The authors are indebted to Ms. H. Flückiger for the preparation of this manuscript.

References

[1] von Schulthess, G. K., E. Ketz, P. A. Schubiger et al.: Regional quantitative noninvasive assessment of cerebral perfusion and function with N-isopropyl-[^{123}I]p-iodoamphetamine. J. Nucl. Med. **26** (1985) 9–16.

[2] Lee R. G. L., T. C. Hill, B. L. Holmann et al.: N-isopropyl(^{123}I)p-iodoamphetamine brain scans with single photon emission tomography: Discordance with transmission tomography. Radiology **145** (1982) 795–799.

[3] Reichmann, K., H. J. Biersack, G. Friedrich et al.: Bedeutung der durch hochenergetische Strahlungskomponenten vom ^{123}J bzw. ^{124}J verursachten Hintergrundstrahlung bei der Hirn-SPECT mit Jod-Amphetamin. Nuc. Compact **6** (1984) 302–304.

[4] von Schulthess, G. K., E. Ketz, A. Bekier: ^{123}I isopropyl-iodoamphetamine (IMP) in the assessment of cerebral perfusion: Is a quantiative noninvasive measurement possible? In "^{123}I Amphetamine," Proceeding of a Colloquium (von Schulthess, G. K. et al., eds.). Editiones Roche, Basle, Switzerland 1984.

[5] Moretti. J. L., S. Askienazi, C. Raynaud et al.: N-isopropyl-^{123}I-p-iodoamphetamine: An agent for brain imaging with single photon emission computed tomography. In: Functional Radionuclide Imaging of the Brain (Magistretti, P. L., ed.). Raven Press, New York 1983.

[6] Büll. H. U., article in this book.

[7] La France, N. D., H. N. Wagner, Jr., R. Whitehouse et al.: Decreased accumulation of isopropyl-iodoamphetamine (^{123}I) in brain tumors, J. Nucl. Med. **22** (1981) 1081–1083.

[8] Magistretti, P., R. Uren, D. Stromer et al.: Emission tomographic scans of cerebral blood flow using ^{123}I iodoamphetamine in epilepsy. In: Proceedings of the Third World Congress of Nuclear Medicine and Biology (Raynaud, C., ed.). Pergamon Press, Oxford 1982. p. 139.

[9] Martin, W. R. W., M. E. Raichle: Cerebellar blood flow and metabolism in cerebral hemisphere infarction. Ann. Neurol. **14** (1983) 168–176.

[10] Shepp, L., B. F. Logan: Fourier reconstruction of a head section. IEEE Trans. Nucl. Sci. NS. **21** (1974) 21–43.

[11] Damasio, H.: A computed tomographic guide to the identification of cerebral vascular territories. Arch. Neurol. **40** (1983) 138–142.

[12] de Leon, M. J., A. E. George, S. M. Ferris et al.: Positron emission computed tomography and computed tomography assessment of the aging human brain. J. Comput. Assist. Tomogr. **8** (1) (1984) 88–94.

Brain SPECT with ^{123}I-Labelled Amphetamine Derivatives in Epilepsy and Migraine

H. J. Biersack. W. Fröscher, H. Penin, P. Bülau, K. Reichmann, C. Winkler

On the basis of positron tomography (PET) results it has been well established that seizures are connected with increases in regional cerebral blood flow and metabolism [1, 7]. In the interictal stage, however, regionally diminished perfusion can be observed in the affected cortical areas [1]. As changes in cerebral function due to seizures are seldom accompanied by structural changes they often cannot be detected by radiographic techniques. Here the EEG is useful, but has significant limitations: It is often difficult to lateralize or localize the origin of the seizure or to assess the severity and extent of underlying cerebral involvement [5]. Since 1982 SPECT with ^{123}I-labelled N-isopropyl amphetamine (IMP) has been used for the evaluation of epilepsy [2–4, 6, 8–13]. By means of this technique, identical findings – ictally increased, interictally decreased tracer accumulation – as with PET were established. In addition, amphetamine SPECT can reveal increased perfusion in epileptic foci at a time when there is focal electrical discharge, even in the absence of clinically recognizable seizures [6]. The present paper presents an overview of our results in a relatively large series of patients with epilepsy. Data are also included of patients with migraine accompagnée – a disease in which EEG pathology may also be observed.

Methods and patients

SPECT of the brain was performed 40–60 minutes after the injection of 6.5 mCi ^{123}I-labelled IMP or N-sec. butyl amphetamine (BMP) provided by Amersham Buchler. A rotating gamma camera (Gammatome T9000/CGR), equipped with a high resolution-low energy collimator, was used for imaging. During one 360° rotation, 64 frames with 4k matrix were acquired within 20 minutes [3]. Transversal, coronal, and sagittal slices were reconstructed within a short processing time, using an array processor. ^{123}I was produced according to the reaction:

$$^{124}_{52}\mathrm{Te}\ (p, 2n)\ ^{123}_{53}\mathrm{I}$$

^{124}I contamination was less than 2%, as the investigations were carried out within 12–13 hours after cyclotron production of the radionuclide.

A total of 50 patients were investigated: 45 patients suffered from epilepsy and 5 from migraine. In all cases the results of cranial computed tomography (CT) as well of EEG examinations were available. In 5 patients nuclear magnetic resonance (NMR) imaging could additionally by performed.

Results

Epilepsy

The results of our investigations are summarized in tables 1–3: Regular SPECT results were obtained in 9 patients, 5 patients showed ictally local increased uptake (figs. 1, 2), and 31 interictally focal decreased uptake (figs. 3, 4). The following results were obtaind regarding the findings of SPECT and CT: In 8 patients CT and SPECT were negative, in 20 cases the same examinations revealed lesions. One patient had a negative SPECT study but showed a CT lesion, and in 16 cases (5 × hyperperfusion, 11 × hypoperfusion) positive SPECT results were obtained despite negative CT. In 20 patients the extent of the lesions – as determined with both techniques – was compared. In 8 patients the extent of lesions detected by SPECT was larger than that found by CT; 2 patients revealed CT lesions larger than the SPECT defects. In 10 patients similar results could be obtained with both techniques. One patient with general cerebral atrophy had a negative amphetamine SPECT.

Migraine

Five patients with migraine were investigated, 3 showed regionally diminished (fig. 5) and 2 regionally increased (fig. 6) uptake. Four of these patients presented EEG signs in the respective cerebral areas.

Discussion

Epilepsy

By means of PET scans, obtained *interictally*, it was possible to reveal dysfunctional brain zones considered responsible for seizures in patients with partial epilepsy. These areas usually appeared normal in CT scans [1]. Our results obtained using SPECT and ^{123}I IMP as a tracer correspond to the above mentioned PET scans. In 11 out of 16 cases with negative CT we found hypoperfusion by means of SPECT. 20 patients with CT-proven lesions showed interictally reduced activity accumulation as well. In 8 of these 20 patients the extent of lesions detected by SPECT was larger than that found by CT. This is well in agreement with the results of Sanabria et al.

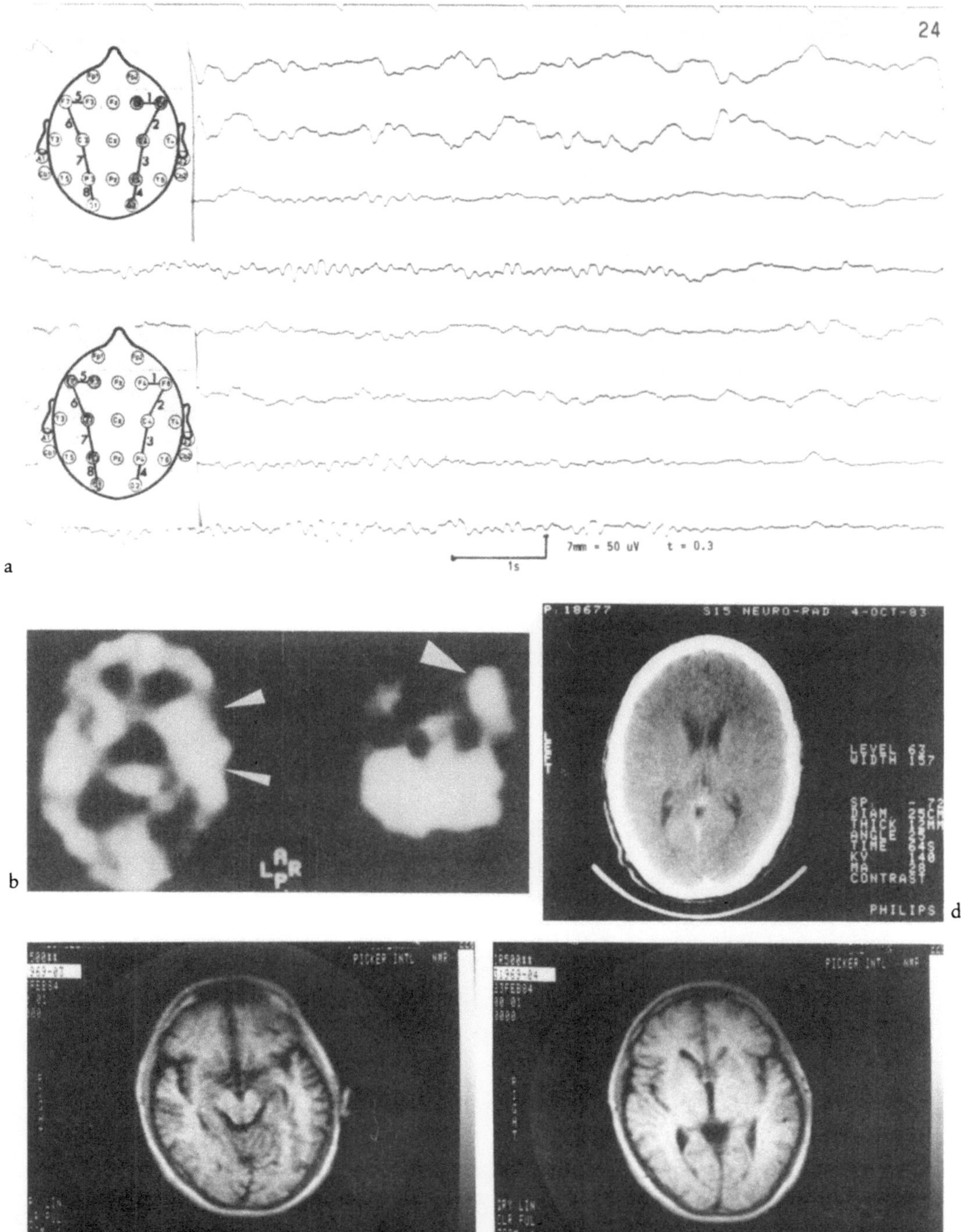

Fig. 1 Epilepsy, right temporal lobe:
a) EEG: focus right temporal lobe; b) Brain SPECT with ^{123}I IMP: increased IMP uptake in the right temporal lobe (ictally); c) NMR: unremarkable; d) CT: unremarkable.

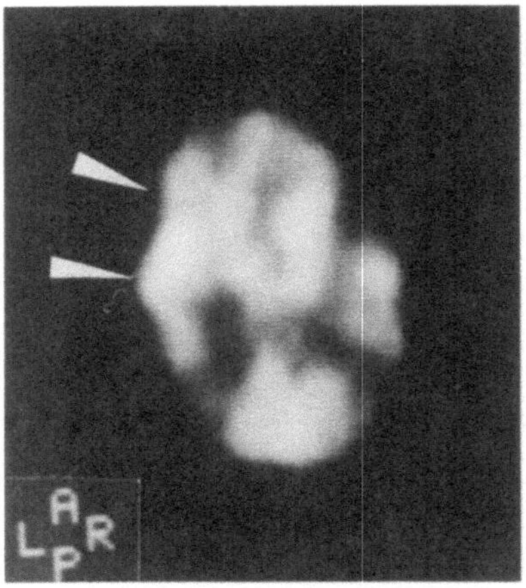

Fig. 2 Ictal IMP-SPECT in epilepsy: increased uptake in the left temporal lobe, according to the EEG focus, but unremarkable CT.

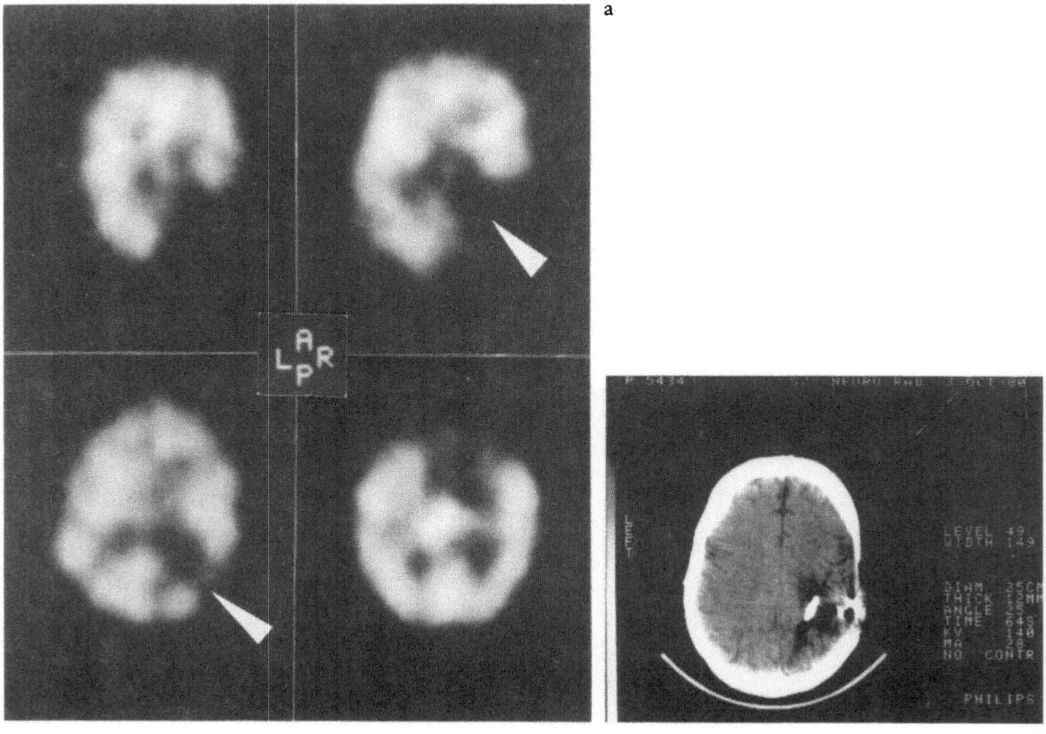

Fig. 3 Symptomatic epilepsy after gunshot wound parieto-occipital right:
a) Brain SPECT with ^{123}I IMP: focally decreased IMP uptake parieto-occipital right; b) CT: lesion parieto-occipital right.

Fig. 4

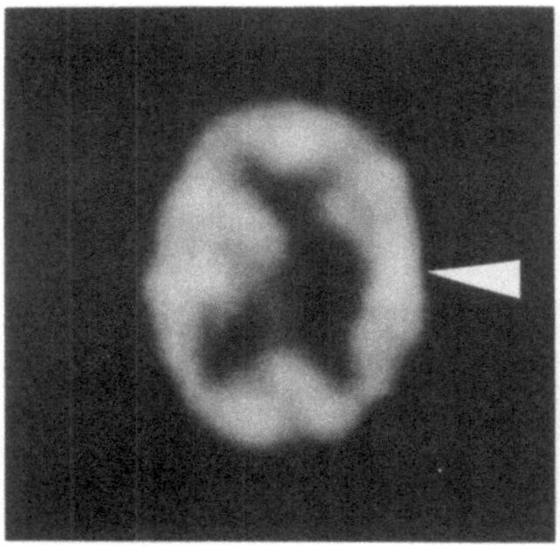

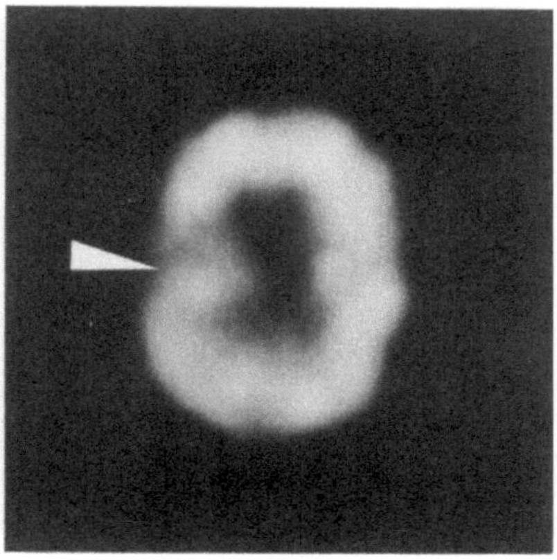

Fig. 5

Fig. 4 Interictal IMP SPECT in epilepsy: descreased uptake in the right temporal lobe, according to the EEG focus, but unremarkable CT.

Fig. 5 IMP SPECT in migraine accompagnée: decreased IMP uptake temporal left, according to the EEG focus.

Table 1 Patients (n = 50)

1. partial epilepsy (n = 45)	
normal SPECT:	9
focal increased uptake:	5
focal decreased uptake:	31
2. migraine (n = 5)	
focal increased uptake:	2
focal decreased uptake:	3

Table 2 Results in partial epilepsy (n = 45)

CT + SPECT normal	8
CT + SPECT abnormal	20*
CT normal/SPECT abnormal	16**
CT abnormal/SPECT normal	1

* in all cases hypoperfusion

** 11 × hypoperfusion (interictal)
5 × hyperperfusion (ictal)

Table 3 Extension of lesions in epilepsy (CT vs SPECT, n = 20)

CT	=	SPECT	n = 10*
SPECT	>	CT	n = 8
SPECT	<	CT	n = 2

* including cerebral atrophy

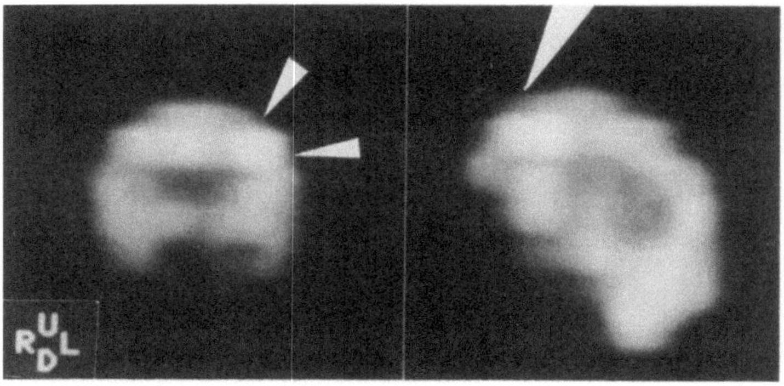

Fig. 6 IMP SPECT in migraine accompagnée: regionally increased IMP uptake frontal left, according to the EEG focus (left: coronar section, right: sagittal section).

[13]. In the *ictal* state PET investigations revealed increased perfusion and metabolism in cortical epileptic foci. The same finding was observed using IMP-SPECT [2, 6, 8, 9, 11, 12]. Five of our patients showed locally increased amphetamine uptake despite negative CT, but they were in accordance with the EEG findings. During the SPECT study all 5 patients presented EEG spike and wave complexes but showed no clinical evidence of seizure. A similar case was described by Holman et al. [6]. Thus, increased perfusion can therefore occur at a time when there is focal electrical discharge but in the absence of clinically recognizable seizures.

From these data it seems obvious that IMP-SPECT plays a significant role in the study of epilepsy, particularly in those patients being considered for surgery (temporal lobectomy), when seizure activity is poorly controlled by medication. Because IMP studies are simple to perform and do not require much patient cooperation, it is relatively easy to study patients in an attempt to localize seizure foci. We have shown that IMP can identify a seizure focus by demonstrating increased regional blood flow in a specific area of the cortex. For this the radiopharmaceutical has to be injected during the seizure or at a time when the patient's EEG shows focal signs. On the other hand, interictally hypoperfused cortial areas might be observed in many cases. Depth electrodes, although valuable in those patients, may not be successful in localizing the primary epileptic focus in every patient [1]. IMP-SPECT, however, can be helpful in detecting the exact focus localization, especially when a secondary onset is propagated at a site distant from the recording depth electrode [1]. It should be stressed that radiographic techniques usually fail to reveal respective foci.

Migraine accompagnée

To date there are no reports dealing with the role of amphetamine SPECT in migraine which might explain our inconsistent observations of regional hyper- (n = 2) or hypoperfusion (n = 3). However, these results suggest that a migraine attack may be accompanied by regional hypoperfusion and consecutive hyperperfusion or vice versa. In four of five cases corresponding focal EEG signs were observed – despite negative CT – suggesting that IMP-SPECT may render possible the differential diagnosis of migraine accompagnée when compared to other types. Moreover, the method may be useful for the evaluation of therapeutic measures.

References

[1] Alavi, A., M. Reivich, S. C. Jones et al.: Functional imaging of the brain with positron emission tomography, in: Nuclear Medicine Annual 1982, ed. by L. M. Freeman and H. Weissmann, Raven Press 1982, p. 319.

[2] Biersack, H. J., H. Penin, K. Reichmann et al.: SPECT of the brain using a rotating gamma camera system and ^{123}I-isopropyl amphetamine: results in epilepsy, in: Neuroimaging, ed. by F. Gerstenbrand, N. Grcevic, and F. Aichner, Gustav Fischer Stuttgart/New York 1984, p. 231.

[3] Biersack, H. J., H. Penin, A. Hartmann et al.: Zerebrale Emissions-Computertomographie (SPECT) mit ^{123}J-markierten Amphetaminen. Dtsch. med. Wschr. **109** (1984) 1155.

[4] Chauvel, P., E. Sanabria, S. Askienazy et al.: Single photon tomography using ^{123}I-N-isopropyl amphetamine in partial epilepsy, in: Epilepsy international Symposium 1983, Abstracts, p. 242.

[5] Fröscher, W.: Untersuchungen zur Konstanz von EEG-Merkmalen bei Epilepsie-Patienten. Zschr. EEG-EMG **13** (1982) 9.

[6] Holman, B. L., T. C. Hill, P. L. Magistretti: Brain imaging with emission computed tomography and radiolabeled amines. Invest. Radiol. **17** (1982) 206.

[7] Kuhl, D. E.: Mapping local cerebral glucose utilization in normal aging and in cerebrovascular, degenerative, and epileptic disorders, in: Positron emission tomography of the brain, ed. by W.-D. Heiss and M. E. Phelps, Springer Berlin/Heidelberg/New York 1983, p. 128.

[8] Magistretti, P., R. Uren, H. Blume et al.: Delineation of epileptic focus by single photon emission tomography. Eur. J. Nucl. Med. **7** (1982) 484.

[9] Magistretti, P., R. Uren, D. Schomer et al.: Emission tomographic scans of cerebral blood flow using ^{123}I iodoamphetamine in epilepsy, in: Proc. III. World Congr. Nucl. Med. & Biol., ed. by C. Raynaud, Pergamon Press 1982, p. 139.

[10] O'Leary, D. H., T. C. Hill, R. G. Lee et al.: The use of ^{123}I-iodoamphetamine and single-photon emission computed tomography to assess local cerebral blood flow. AJNR **4** (1983) 547.

[11] Podreka, I., K. Höll, P. Dal-Bianco et al.: Anwendungsgebiete von ^{123}J-Amphetamin (IMP) Studien in der Neurologie, in: Radioaktive Isotope in Klinik und Forschung, Bd. 16/I. hrsg. v. R. Höfer u. H. Bergmann. Egermann, Wien 1984, S. 1.

[12] Podreka, I., B. Mamoli, P. Dal-Bianco et al.: EEG and SPECT brain studies with N-isopropyl-^{123}I-p-iodoamphetamine in patients with epileptic seizures. Third Europ. Conf. of EEG and clinical neurophysiology, Basle, Sept. 1983, Abstract p. 83.

[13] E. Sanabria, P. Chauvel, S. Askienazy et al.: Single photon emission computed tomography (SPECT) using ^{123}I-isopropyl-iodo-amphetamine (IAMP) in partial epilepsy, in: Cerebral Blood Flow, Metabolism, and Epilepsy, Proc. Int. Symp., Montpellier, June 1983, ed. by M. Baldy-Moulinier, D. H. Ingvar, and B. S. Meldrum. John Libbey Eurotext London/Paris 1983, p. 82.

IMP-SPECT and Amino Acid-PET in Brain Tumors

O. Schober, G. J. Meyer, H. Creutzig, H. Hundeshagen

The increased metabolic activity of rapidly growing tissue has become a target for measurements with positron emission tomography (PET), which has been proven to be a sensitive tool for the assessment of local brain function in both, normal and pathological states [8, 12, 16, 27, 30].

There was a positive correlation between glucose (2-fluoro-2-deoxy-D-glucose: ^{18}F-FDG) uptake in gliomas and their histological grade [8], whereas cerebellar glucose metabolism is depressed on the contralateral side [27, 30]. In addition there is evidence to suggest that in primary brain tumors glucose is metabolized anaerobically. Tumor regional cerebral blood flow is comparable to that in the contralateral cortex, whereas regional cerebral oxygen consumption is depressed in tumor tissue. Glucose extraction ratios are similiar for tumor and brain tissue [30].

Very recently attempts have made by Bustany et al. [4]. Phelps et al. [28], and Meyer et al. [24] to set up and analyse quantitative kinetic models for the determination of protein synthesis in brain tissue. However, because of the complexicitiy of the model, metabolic turnover rates of brain protein synthesis have not been determined quantitatively up to now. Nevertheless uptake ratios of amino acids may prove useful for both, the semiquantitative understanding of the biochemical process "in vivo" and the clinical need for differential diagnosis.

^{11}C-labeled amino acids, DL-valine and DL-tryptophane have been used to image brain tumors [11]. In a case report Bergström et al. [1] demonstrated discrepancies in a brain tumor extent as shown by CT and PET using ^{68}Ga-EDTA, ^{11}G-glucose and the non-racemic ^{11}C-L-methionine.

In our own studies methionine was choosen as the amino acid because it is known from "in vitro studies" [34] and from nutritional support (Gadisseux et al., 1984), that methionine exhibits the highest tumor to non-tumor (T/NT) ratios in gliomas and metastatic brain tumors. According to Oldendorf [26] methionine has also a high extraction rate in brain, and finally the routine production of optically pure ^{11}C-labeled stereoisomers imposed no problems.

The mechanism of IMP brain uptake has been discussed in detail [16, 18, 37]. In brain tumors there was no IMP uptake in the early nor in the late scans, regardless of tumor type, perfusion rate or blood brain barrier (BBB) damage [6]. In a prospective study these findings should be correlated to PET-scans.

Table 1 ^{11}C-Methionine uptake in Positron Emission Tomography (PET): In reconstructed slices which contained no tumor tissue according to the final diagnosis, the left to right hemisphere ratio was 1.0 ± 0.09 SD (n = 50). T/NT: tumor/non-tumor; T/NT: ↓ 0.7–0.9, ∅ 0.9–1.2, ↑ 1.3–1.5, ↑ ↑ 1.6–2.0, ↑ ↑ ↑ >2.0.
Blood Brain Barrier damage (BBS) was verified by Scintigraphy (^{99m}TC-DTPA)[1] or CT with contrast medium[2].

No	Diagnosis	T/NT Ratio	BBB Damage
1	Astrocytoma II	↑	∅ [1,2]
2	metast. brain tumor (partly necrotic)	↑	++ [2]
3	metast. brain tumor	↑ ↑	+ [1,2]
4	glioblastoma	↑ ↑	+ [2]
5	Astrocytoma IV	↑ ↑ ↑	+++ [2]
6	meningeoma	↑ ↑	+++ [2]
7	calcified microangioma	∅	+ [1,2]
8	infarction	↓	+ [1,2]
9	infarction	↓	+ [1,2]

Patients and methods

Tomographic imaging was performed on 7 patients with brain tumors prior to surgery and in 2 patients with stroke (tab. 1). None of the invididuals had undergone chemical or radiation therapy before. All patients gave informed consent to the following protocol.

The patients received about 5 mCi of N-isopropyl ^{123}I-p-iodoamphetamine (^{123}I-(p,5n)-IMP). The radiochemical purity averaged 94%, the waiting time to scan was 10 min for the early scan. Late scan were performed 3.5–6 h p.i. The camera head (Siemens ZLC 3700) with a high resolution collimator was as close to the head of the patients as possible. Data aquisition was obtained by in 64 projections (64 × 64 matrix) for 20 sec per projection. Image reconstruction was performed in a MDS-A-3 system by filtered back projection and a medium Hanning window. Slice thickness is 2 voxel, corresponding to 12 mm.

The preparation and quality control of ^{11}C-L-methionine is described elsewhere [22, 23]. The optical purity of the isomer was controlled by analysis of the product by circular dichroism and polarimetry. Both methods confirmed that the L-form is obtained in >90% purity. The racemization under physiological solvent conditions is negligible.

About 20 mCi of ^{11}C-L-methionine were injected intravenously. 10 min after the injection the patient was positioned under the positron camera (Model 4200 Cycl. Corp.) in supine position, and a 20 min recording of the head was performed [5, 32].

The data were analyzed on a PDP 11/55 computer system. Absorption correction was carried out with ellipse phantom calculations. Up to 10 slices with a thickness of about 15–18 mm were reconstructed. All data presented here are treated for relative uptake of tumor to non-tumor regions in the brain.

The CT scans were obtained with a GE 9800 instrument. Intravenous contrast material (Rayvist^{TM}) was used as indicated. Section thickness was 10 mm.

The results of the PET and IMP tomograms were compared and correlated in 5 of 9 patients to the findings of conventional ^{99m}Tc-DTPA-scan and angiography.

Results

All primary and malignant brain tumors as well as the infarcted regions did not take up IMP (fig. 1). The investigated tumors showed defects ranging from 10–50% when compared with the contralateral side, in the early scan as well as in the late scan.

All methionine uptake data in slices containing tumor tissue are summarized in table 1. The uptake of methionine increased with the malignancy of the tumor with the highest ratio of 2.6 in an astrocytoma IV. In a meningeoma a high methione uptake was observed in the tumor, but not in the surrounding edema. In the two stroke patients we found a diminished methionine uptake.

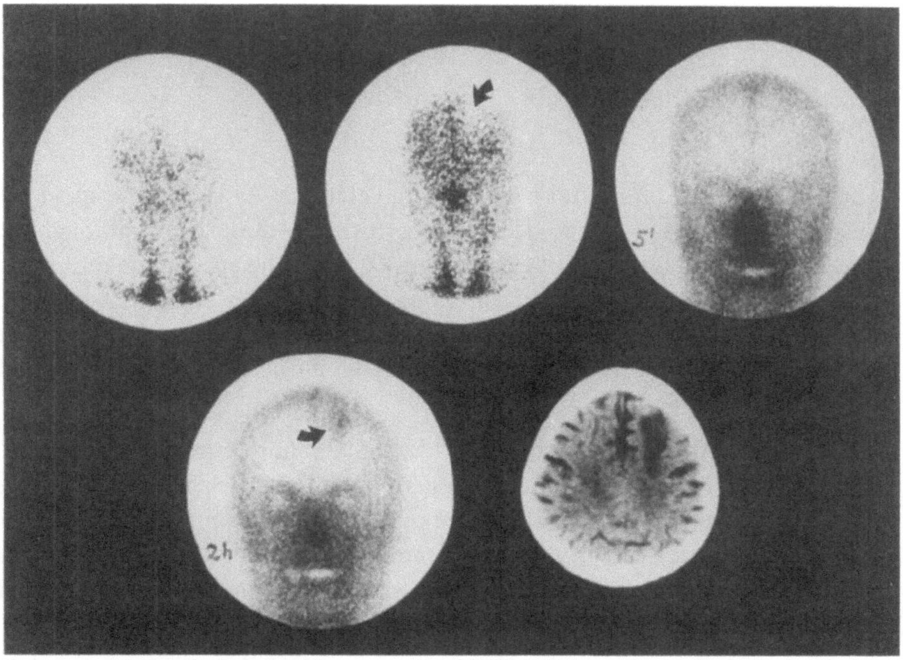

Fig. 1 A patient with a stroke has a positive conventional ^{99m}Tc-DTPA scan in the planar image. During the perfusion phase (arrow) a diminished activity is visualized. The corresponding CT finding demonstrates the defect as well, while in the PET study a diminished ^{11}C-L-methionine uptake was noticed.

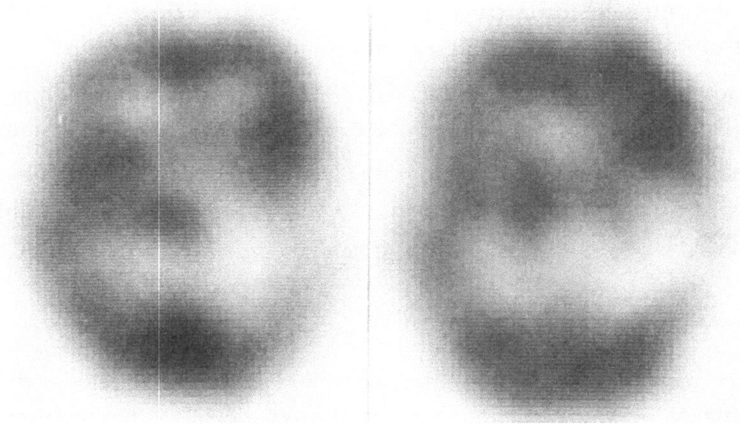

a b

Fig. 2a, b In brain tumors, as in the astrocytoma III, there was no ^{123}I-IMP uptake in the early (10–35 min p.i.) as well as in the late (4 h p.i.) (transversal) scans. In the cortex region is some "filling in" noticed.

In five patients conventional ^{99m}Tc-DTPA scans were performed in order to investigate the blood brain barrier (BBB). Two patients with a positive ^{99m}Tc scan accumulated no or only very small amounts of ^{11}C-methionine, while the patient with the astrocatoma II, who showed no ^{99m}Tc-DTPA uptake, had a positive ^{11}C-methionine accumulation. The two stroke patients showed a positive ^{99m}Tc-DTPA scan (fig. 2).

Discussion

The brain tumors did not take up iodoamphetamine. As Holman et al. [10] stated, this may be related in part to decreased perfusion in these areas, although the most likely explanation is that tumor tissue does not have the appropiate receptor sites or metabolic pathways to permit retention of the radiotracer at the time of imaging. In some of these cases, normal or increased vascularity of the tumor is seen at angiography. In cerebrovascular disease the diminished uptake may reflect decreased perfusion [3, 6, 21].

When compared with other amino acids, the amount of free methionine in brain tissue is small. However the uptake of methionine in single pass extraction measurements is relatively high and is surpassed only by phenylalanine, leucine, and tyrosine [31]. This indicates a high utilisation rate of methionine which should make it a suitable tracer for protein synthesis. A recent comparison by of ten amino acids for tumor uptake confirmed the high uptake of methionine [14].

Having left the plasma, methionine may enter two different reaction pathways. It may be activated for protein synthesis by aminoacyl-tRNA-synthease and ATP or may be activated by ATP yielding S-adenosyl-methionine which undergoes subsequent degradation. With ^{11}C-labeled methionine labeled in the S-methyl position, difficulties may arise from transmethylation reactions [24]. Because these reactions occur not only in brain tissue but take place in the rest of the body, and especially in the liver, the plasma pool also becomes contaminated with other tracers. For the quantitative measurement of protein synthesis rates, it is therefore necessary to control the plasma constituents or to label methionine in the 1-carboxyl position, and to include the CO-2 pool in the compartment model [4, 24, 28].

However, as long as no absolute quantitative data are derived from the measurements, the transmethylation reactions which account for only a small fraction in brain tissue, may be neglected.

Amino acids may enter the brain by different uptake mechanisms. With an intact blood brain barrier (BBB), the main transport of amino acids into brain tissue is carrier facilitated [19, 25]. Any increased uptake due to this mechanism could be related to enhanced metabolic activity of the tissue.

Slight moderate damage to the BBB can result in an inhibition of the transport system and a diminished uptake of the tracer, while a higher degree of damage may leed to a free diffusible uptake [35]. The carrier mediated uptake can be suppressed also by overloading of the carrier system with competing substrates.

The remaining diffusible uptake is flow limited, as can be expected, according to the model by Renkin and Crone [7, 29] (E = exp (-PxS/F); E: extraction; PxS: permeability surface-area product; F: flow). Nevertheless, decreased perfusion does not necessarily lead to increased uptake due to enhanced extraction, because the uptake is a product of vascularisation and extraction, and remains unpredictable in most patholocigal cases.

While soft tissue tumors have been reported to exhibit both, enhanced perfusion and concomittant glutamate uptake [13], cerebral tumors have only slightly changed perfusion when compared with the unaffected tissue on the contralateral side [20, 32, 36].

Because usually the diffusive uptake is a relative slow process and typically BBB breakdown can be visualized in ^{99m}Tc-DTPA scans in late images only, the present findings which were obtained within 30 min after injection, seem to refer to an active metabolic process. The strongest support for this interpretation stems from the observation that in two cases the positive ^{99m}Tc-scan was accompanied by no or only slight ^{11}C-methionine uptake, while an astrocytoma II with no BBB damage showed a distinct methionine uptake. In infarctions with BBB breakdown the methionine uptake was insignificant.

A similiar finding was reported by the NIH group in ^{18}F-FDG uptake studies for CNS tumors [8]. In this study a correlation wa found for uptake and tumor grade also with mismatch of CT contrast enhancement – due to BBB disrupture – and ^{18}F-FDG uptake.

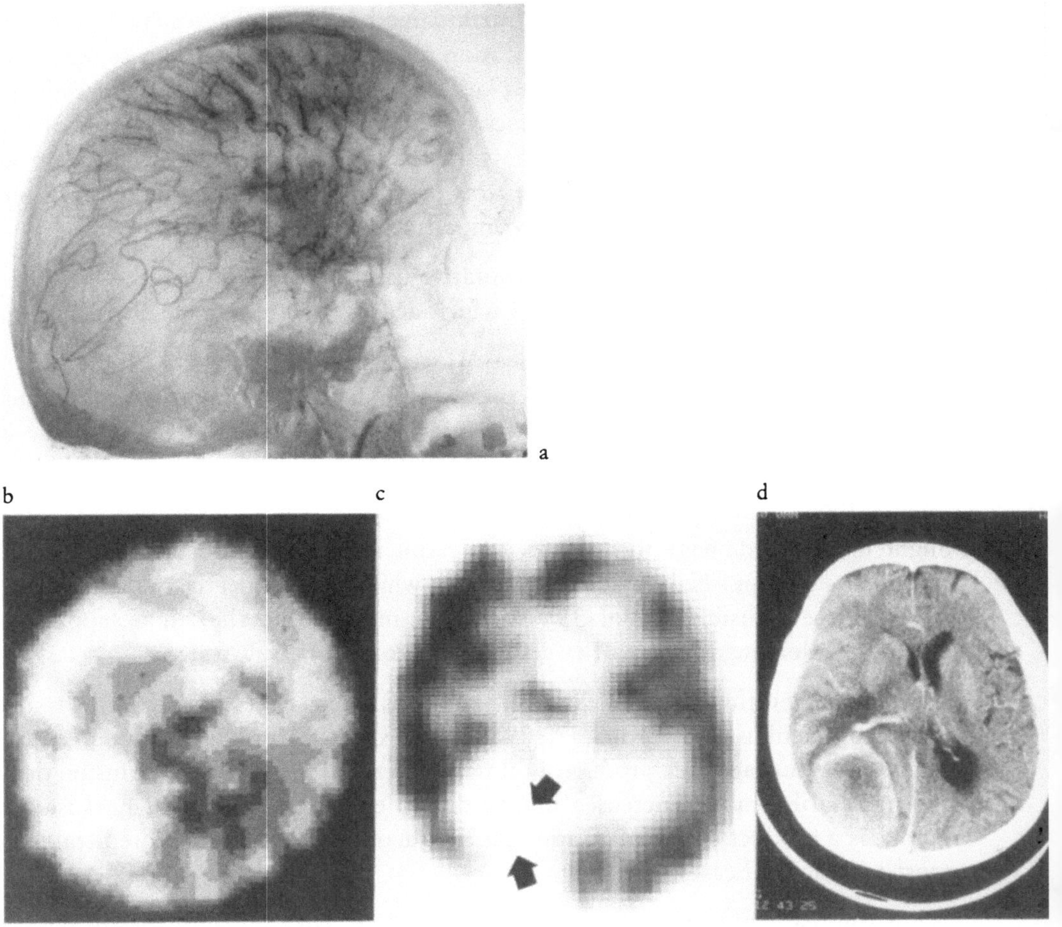

Fig. 3a, b, c, d The IMP study of a patient with metastasis in the occipital lobe shows diminished uptake (arrow) in the corresponding region (c). The carotid angiography (a) shows tumors signs, i.e. stretching of the vessels. The X-ray CT (d) scan obtained on the day after the PET (b) study shows the tumor in the right occipital lobe with ringlike enhancement after contrast medium. The necrosis in the center of the tumor was proven histologically. The PET study with ^{11}C-L-methionine shows a tumor/contralateral non-tumor ratio of 1.9 in the more lateral part of the tumor. Only this part of the tumor is visualized positively.

Conclusion

In brain tumors there was no IMP uptake in the early scan as well as in the late scans, regardless of the tumor type, perfusion rate or blood brain barrier damage. In brain tumor this may reflect diminished receptor sites for IMP.

Although a contribution to the uptake of ^{11}C-methionine in brain tumors by BBB damage can not be ruled out from the current data, the missing uptake in proven

BBB damage cases indicates that the amount of contribution by diffusive processes is relatively small. Our clinical data support the suggestion that there is a correlation of methionine uptake with the tumor grade in astrocytomas.

References

[1] Bergström, M., V. P. Collins, E. Ehrin et al.: Case Report: Discrepancies in Brain Tumor Extent as Shown by Computed Tomography and Positron Emission Tomography using (^{68}Ga)EDTA, (^{11}C)Glucose, and (^{11}C)Methionine. J. Comp. Assist. Tomogr. 7 (1983) 1062-1066.

[2] Biersack, H. J., A. Hartmann, G. Friedrich et al.: Zur Ursache der gekreuzten zerebellaren Diaschisis bei zerebrovaskulären Erkrankungen. Nucl. Med. **23** (1984) 227–230.

[3] Büll, U., E. Kleinhans, K. Schmiedek et al.: Relativbestimmung von Hemisphärendurchblutung. Nucl. Med. **23** (1984) 247–252.

[4] Bustany, P., J. E. Henry, T. Sargent et al.: Local brain protein metabolism in dementia and schizophrenia: in vivo studies with ^{11}C-methionine and positron emission tomography. In: Positron Emission Tomography of the Brain (Heiss, W. D., Phelps, M. E., eds.) pp. 208–211. Springer, Berlin 1983.

[5] Carrol, L. R.: Design and performance characteristics of a production model positron imaging system. IEEE Trans. Nucl. Sci. **25** (1978) 606–614.

[6] Creutzig, H., O. Schober, P. Gielow et al.: Cerebral dynamics of N-Isopropyl.(^{123}I)p-Iodoamphetamine. J. Nucl. Med., in press (1985).

[7] Crone, C.: The permeability of capillaries in various organs as determined by use of the indicator discussion method. Acta Physiol. Scand. **58** (1963) 292–305.

[8] DiChiro, G., R. L. DelaPaz, R. A. Brooks et al.: Glucose utilization of cerebral gliomas measured by (^{18}F)fluorodeoxyglucose and positron emission tomography. Neurology (NY) **32** (1982) 1323–1329.

[9] Gadisseux, P., J. D. Ward, H. F. Young et al.: Nutrition and the neurosurgical patient J. Neurosurg. **60** (1984) 219–232.

[10] Holman, B. L., T. C. Hill, R. G. L. Lee et al.: Brain Imaging with Radiolabeled Amins. Nucl. Med. Ann. 1983. Freeman, L. M., Weissman, H. S., eds. Raven Press, New York 1983.

[11] Hübner, K. F., J. T. Purvis, S. M. Mahaley et al.: Brain Tumor Imaging by Positron Emission Computed Tomography Using ^{11}C-Labeled Amino Acids. J. Comp. Assist. Tomogr. **6** (1982) 544–550.

[12] Jones, T.: Positron Emission Tomography in the Study of Tumors. Sem. Nucl. Med. **15**, in press (1985).

[13] Knapp, W. H., F. Helus, H. Sinn et al.: N-13-glutamate uptake in malignancy: Its relationship to blood flow. J. Nucl. Med. **25** (1984) 989–997.

[14] Kubota, K., K. Yamada, H. Fukada et al.: Tumor detection with carbon-11-labelled amino acids. Eur. J. Nucl. Med. **9** (1984) 136–140.

[15] Kuhl, D. E., J.-L. Barrio, S. C. Huang et al.: Quantifying local cerebral blood flow by N-isopropyl-(^{123}I) p-iodoamphetamine (IMP) tomography, J. Nucl. Med. **23** (1983) 196–203.

[16] Kuhl, D. E.: Mapping Local Cerebral Glucose Utilization in Normal Aging and in Cerebrovascular, Degenerative, and Epileptic Disorders. In: Positron Emission Tomography of the Brain (Heiss, W. D., Phelps, M. E., eds.) pp. 128–138. Springer, Berlin, Heidelberg, New York 1983.

[17] Kushner, M., A. Alavi, M. Reivich et al.: Contralateral Cerebellar Hypometabolism Following Cerebral Insult: A Positron Emission Tomography Study. Ann. Neurol. **15** (1984) 425–434.

[18] Lafrance, N. D., H. N. Wagner, jr., R. Whitehouse et al.: Decreased accumulation of isopropyl-iodoamphetamine (^{123}I) in brain tumors. J. Nucl. Med. **22** (1981) 1081–1083.

[19] Lajtha, A. J. Toth: The brain barrier system. V: Stereospecificity of amino acid uptake, exchange and efflux, J. Neurochem. 10 (1963) 909–920.
[20] Lammertsma, A. A., R. S. J. Wise, J. D. Heather et al.: Correction for the presence of intravascular oxygen-15 in the steady-state technique for measuring regional oxygen extraction ratio in the brain. 2: Results in normal subjects and brain tumor and stroke patients. J. Cerebr. Blood. Flow. Metabol. 3 (1983) 425–431.
[21] Lee, R. G. L., T. C. Hill, B. L. Holman et al.: N-Isopropyl(^{123}I)p-Iodoamphetamine Brain Scans with Single-Phton Emission Tomography: Discordance with Transmission Computed Tomography. Radiology **145** (1982) 795–799.
[22] Meyer, G.-J., A. Osterholz, H. Hundeshagen: Routine Production and Quality Control of ^{11}C-methionine. J. Labeled. Comp. Radiopharm. **19** (1982) 1286–1287.
[23] Meyer, G.-J., A. Osterholz, H. Hundeshagen: Routine Quality Control of ^{11}C-labeled Radiopharmaceuticals by HPLC. J. Radioanalyt. Chem. **80** (1983) 229–235.
[24] Meyer, G.-J., O. Schober, H. Hundeshagen: Uptake of ^{11}C-L-methionine and D-methionine in brain tumors. Eur. J. Nucl. Med. **10** (1985) 373–376.
[25] Neame, K. D.: A comparison of the transport systems for amino acids in brain, intestine, kidney, and tumor. In. Brain Barrier Systems (Lajtha, A., Ford, D. H., eds.). pp. 357–366. Elsevier Publ. Comp., Amsterdam 1968.
[26] Oldendorf, W.: Clearance of radiolabeled substances by brain after arterial injection using a diffusible standard. In: Research Methods in Neurochemistry (Marks, N., Rodnight, R., eds.,). pp. 91–112. Plenum. New York 1981.
[27] Patronas, N. J., G. DiChiro, B. H. Smith et al.: Depressed cerebellar glucose metabolism in supratentorial tumors. Brain Res. **291** (1984) 93–101.
[28] Phelps, M. E., J. R. Barrio, S. C. Huang et at.: Criteria for tracer kinetic measurement of cerebral protein synthesis in man with positron computed tomography. Ann. Neurol. **15** Suppl. (1984) 192–202.
[29] Renkin, E. M.: Transport of potassium-42 from blood to tissue in isolated mammalian skeletal muscle. Amer. J. Physiol. **197** (1959) 1205–1210.
[30] Rhodes. C. G., R. S. J. Wise, J. M. Gibbs et al.: In Vivo Disturbance of the Oxidative Metabolism of Glucose in Human Cerebral Gliomas. Ann. Neurol. **14** (1983) 614–626.
[31] Roberts, S.: Influence of elevated circulating levels of amino acids on cerebral concentraction and utilization of amino acids. In: Brain Barrier Systems (Lajtha, A., Ford, D. H., eds.) pp. 235–243. Elsevier Publ. Comp., Amsterdam 1968.
[32] Schober, O., G.-J. Meyer, C. Bossaler et al: Quantitative Determination of Regional Extravascular Lung Water and Regional Blood Volume in Congestive Heart Failure. Eur. J. Nucl. Med. **10** (1985) 17–24.
[33] Schober, O., G.-J. Meyer, D. Stolke et al.: Brain Tumor Imaging Using ^{11}C-Labeled L-Methionine and D-Methionine. J. Nucl. Med. **26** (1985) 98–99.
[34] Shibasaki, T., J. Uki, T. Kanoh et al.: Composition of free amino acids in brain tumors. Acta Neurol. Scandinav. **60** (1979) 301–311.
[35] Steinwall, O.: Transport inhibition phenomena in unilateral chemical injury of blood brain barrier. In: Brain Barrier Systems (Lajtha, A., Ford, D. H., eds.) pp. 357–366. Elsevier Publ. Comp., Amsterdam 1968.
[36] Walker, M. D., ed.: Research Issues in Positron Emission Tomography. Ann. Neurol. **15** Suppl. (1984).
[37] Winchell, H. S., W. D. Horst, L. Braun et al.: N-isoprophyl-(^{123}I)p-iodoamphetamine: single pass brain uptake and washout; binding to brain synaptosomes, and localization in dog and monkey brain. J. Nucl. Med. **21** (1980) 947–951.

Acknowledgments

The authors thank Dr. P. Gielow for preparing the ^{123}I-IMP, Drs. H. J. Helmecke and D. Junker of the cyclotron group, and Dr. H. Becker and Prof. Dr. Dr. H. Dietz, and their patients for their cooperation.

^{123}I-p-iodo-Isopropyl Amphetamine for Brain Tumor Diagnosis

J. L. Moretti, S. Askienazy, C. Raynaud, A. Sergent, P. Cesaro, M. Tardy

Brain tumors were routinely delineated on current planar scintigraphy by accumulation of hydrophilic compounds like Technetium derivatives due to their increased blood-brain barrier (BBB) permeability. Winchell introduced a new lipophilic agent, p-iodo-isopropyl amphetamine ^{123}I (IAMP), with a high affinity to normal brain tissue [1]. Following a short survey on four astrocytomas done by N. D. Lafrance [2]; we applied IAMP tomoscintigraphy to a group of 27 proven brain tumors of various grades and natures, compared its results with CT scan and ^{99m}Tc scintigraphy.

Materials and methods

^{123}I-IAMP was prepared according to an exchange reaction published elsewhere [3, 4] using a commercial kit (CIS, France). Purity control was achieved by silica gel chromatography and the labelling yield was 98.28 ± 0.86% (n : 25 ± sd). An amount of 2–7 mCi (74–259 MBq) of IAMP ^{123}I per 10 mg of IAMP was injected to our patients, depending on the type of device used.

Most of our studies were performed using iodine produced by the ^{124}Te (p, 2n) ^{123}I, containing less than 4% of ^{124}I as impurity.

γ Tomoscintigraphy was obtained using two types of SPECT systems – a detector array system and a rotating γ Camera.

The detector array, TOMOMATIC 64[1], provides brain transverse sections with high sensitivity [5]. Accumulating for 5 mm after multiple rotation, the counting rate per slice was 300.000 counts. Spatial resolution in the reconstructed plane was 1.7 cm (FWHM). Three different rotating camera systems were used in this study, one General Electric camera (GE 400) connected to a SIMIS 3[2], and two Gammatomes[2], one of which was connected to an ADAC computer and the other to a SIMIS 3.

The data were accumulated by the rotating cameras during 40 minutes and upon 64 angles providing three to five million counts. Such an accumulation was beginning

[1] Produced by Medimatic Inc., Gersonsvej 7, 2900 Hellerup, Denmark.

[2] Produced by Sopha Medical, Av. de Scandinavie, B.P. 81, 92940 Les Ullis, France.

20 minutes after intravenous injection into patients who has their eyes closed. The filtered back-projection (FBP) method was used for image reconstruction.

Patients

Primary tumors were investigated in 20 patients including 13 astrocytomas, 3 glioblastomas and 4 oligodendrogliomas.

Secondary tumors were explored in 5 patients with metastasis. Two meningiomas were also explored.

Results of brain tomoscintigraphy was then compared to CT scans and ^{99m}Tc planar scintigraphy results.

Results

Brain tumors were detected very easily by a lack of activity in the tumor in all but two equivocal cases (low grade astrocytomas). The lack of IAMP tumor accumulation was irrespective of grade and BBB permeability as observed with ^{99m}Tc scintigraphy and positive contrast CT scan. As demonstrated on table 1, the sensitivity of IAMP ^{123}I was 88%, versus 100% for CT scan and only 31% for ^{99m}Tc scintigraphy.

Table 1 Compared results of ^{99m}Tc scintigraphy, CT scan and ^{123}I-I AMP brain tomoscintigraphy on brain tumors

Number of cases	Pathology	^{99m}Tc	CT	^{123}I-I AMP
13	Astrocytoma	10−	13+	13+
		1+		
3	Glioblastoma	1+	3+	3+
4	Oligodendroglioma	2+	4+	3+
		1−		1−
2	Meningioma	−	2+	2+
5	Metastasis	2+	4+	3+
		1−		2−
27	positive results	31%	100%	88%

Discussion

Tab. 1 demonstrated a very low score for brain tumor detectability by conventional ^{99m}Tc scintigraphy. This bad unusual score was due to a large number of low grade astrocytomas. Most authors postulate that IAMP brain uptake is due to the affinity for high capacity, relatively non specific binding sites for amines and that brain distribution is related to local blood flow, how can one explain the lack of IAMP uptake in high vascularized tumors like glioblastomas and moreover, a lack of activity in very low grade astrocytomas? One can postulate that the removal of this monoamine from circulation is achieved through the podocytes into glial cells. Astrocytes are known to have high affinity for Noradrenaline [5] and possess GABA [6] binding sites.

Does p-Iodo-isopropyl amphetamine accumulate into normal astrocyte? To answer this question; astroglial cells obtained from new born mouse brain hemispheres and grown until maturation in primary cultures accumulated IAMP in a linear mode from a media containing 1–10 μM of the substrate for at least 5 mn at 37 °C. Kinetics studies were performed by measuring the uptake at 10 different concentrations during 3 minutes. Results were obtained by substracting the radioactivity value at 0 °C under the same conditions, since at that temperature residual transport probably corresponds to a simple diffusion process. Graphic analysis showed the presence of a saturable uptake system in astrocytes with a Km of 20 ± 5 μM and a V_{MAX} of 500 ± 50 p.mol/min/mg of cell proteins (mean value from 3 different experiments) [7].

Does tumorous astrocytes have lost this ability to accumulate p-iodo-amphetamine event when their perfusion is important? Is flow without binding sites equivalent to poor extraction? Authors have described the biochemical alterations of tumorous astrocytes as, a low oxydative metabolism an increase of aerobic glycolysis [8] and plyamines formation [9] ability to thrive without oxygen and carbohydrate supply [10]. In these abnormal astrocytes, GABA pathway is not functional [11] adenylate cyclase is low [12], there are few steroid receptors [13] and glial fibrillary protein is abnormal [14].

The lower activity seen in our investigated tumors may be related to a lack of binding sites permitting quicker washout. This impaired extraction efficiency of IAMP by tumorous tissue more deeply deserves further explanations.

According to our results, ^{123}I-IAMP SPECT was not the best method for brain tumor localization, but it delineated the extension of tumoral lesions in deep structures such as thalamic nuclei or basal ganglia. These low activity areas were well delineated on frontal and sagittal slices when using rotating cameras, thus faciliting the spotting of stereotactic biopsies.

References

[1] Winchell, H.S., W.D. Horst, L. Braun et al.: N-isopropyl(^{123}I)p-iodoamphetamine: single pass brain uptake and washout; binding to brain synaptosomes; and localization in dog and monkey brain. J. Nucl. Med. **21** (1980) 947–952.

[2] Lafrance, N.D., H.N. Wagner, P. Whitehouse et al.: Decreased accumulation of isopropyl-Iodoamphetamine (^{123}I) in brain tumors. J. Nucl. Med. **22** (1981) 1081–1083.

[3] Moretti, J. L., S. Askienazy, C. Raynaud et al.: La N-Isopropyl-p-Iodoamphétamine ^{123}I en tomoscintigraphie cérébrale. Ann. Radiol. **26** (1983) 59.
[4] Moretti, J. L., S. Askienazy, C. Raynaud et al.: N-Isopropyl-^{123}I-p-Iodoamphetamine: an agent for brain imaging with single-photon emission computerized tomography. In: Functional Radionuclide Imaging of the brain (ed. by P. L. Magistretti). Raven Press, pp. 231–246. New York 1983.
[5] Su, Y. F., L. Cubeddu, J. P. Perkins: Regulation of adenosine 3′5′ monophosphate content of human astrocytoma cells: desentisization to catecholamines and prostaglandins. J. Cyclic Nucleotide Res. **2** (1976) 257–270.
[6] Hamberger, A., L. Svennerholm: Composition of gangliosides and phospholipids of neuronal and glial cell enriched fractions. J. Neurochem. **18** (1971) 1821–1829.
[7] Tardy, M., C. Fages: Unpublished data U 282 INSERM (1985).
[8] Warburg, O.: The metabolism of tumors. In: Investigations from the Kaiser Wilhelm Institute for Biology, Berlin-Dahlem (ed. by O. Warburg, trans. by F. Dickens). Constable and Co. Ltd., London 1930.
[9] Kremzner, L. T.: Polyamine metabolism in normal and neoplastic neural tissue. In: Polyamines in normal and neoplastic growth (ed. by D. H. Russell). Raven Press, pp. 27–40, New York 1973.
[10] Greenstein, J. P.: Chemistry of tumors. In: Biochemistry of Cancer, Academic Press, pp. 327–506, New York 1954.
[11] Allen, N.: Respiration and oxidative metabolism of brain tumors. In: The experimental biology of tumors (ed. by. W. M. Kirsch, E. C. Paoletti, P. Paoletti et al.) Springfield, III, pp. 243–274, 1972.
[12] Furman, M. A., K. Schulman: Cyclic AMP and adenyl cyclase in brain tumors. J. Neurosurg. **46** (1977) 477–483.
[13] Duffy, P. E.: Astrocytes, Normal, Reactive and Neoplastic. Raven Press 1983.
[14] Duffy, P. E., Y. Y. Huang, M. M. Rapport: The relationship of glial fibrillary acidic protein to the shape, motility, and differentiation of human astrocytoma cells. Exp. Cell Res. **139** (1982) 145–157.

An Early Appraisal of Clinical Results of ^{123}I HIPDM-SPECT Studies

V. Di Piero, P. Gerundini, G. L. Lenzi, A. Savi, F. Triulzi, A. Del Maschio, F. Fazio

N,N,N'-trimethyl-N'-(2-hydroxy-3-methyl-5-(^{123}I)-iodobenzyl)-1,3-propanediamine 2 HCl (^{123}I HIPDM) is a lipophilic non charged tracer suitable for tomographic assessment of regional cerebral blood flow (rCBF) [1, 2]. This molecule has been utilized in the assessment of rCBF with single photon emission computerized tomography (SPECT) in patients with neurological disorders [3]. The present report summarizes clinical results obtained so far in a total of 115 tomographic studies from 72 patients with neurological diseases. Clinical subgroups are: 34 Strokes, 22 Reversible Ischemic Attacks, 8 Brain Tumors, 4 Epilepsies and 4 Cranial Trauma.

A standardized protocol was used such as follows: all subjects were premedicated with sodium perclorate solution, to block the thyroid. They were given an intravenous injection of 7–8 mCi of ^{123}I HIPDM, while lying supine, eyes closed, in a quiet and dimmed room. About thirty minutes after injection the brain SPECT study was started, followed by planar images in five views. The SPECT study was performed by rotating the gamma camera around the patient and recording 64 angular views on the computer, using a 64 × 64 matrix.

Approximately 4 million total head counts were recorded for a complete rotation lasting 30 to 50 minutes. We used a commercial rotating gamma camera (General Electric 400 AC) equipped with a low energy, medium resolution parallel hole collimator and dedicated STAR Data General computer. All SPECT data were subsequently reconstructed and attenuation corrected obtaining a complete set of tomographic slices.

Transaxial reconstruction were obtained summing the contents oft wo adjacent pixels, and the center-to-center distance of each slice from a reference plane was 0.64 cm. The orbito-meatal (OM) line was the reference plane for horizontal slices.

Resolution in tomographic plane was 2.3 cm FWHM and slice thickness was 2.3 cm FWHM for one slice; summing two adjacent pixels, slice thicknes was 2.5 cm FWHM.

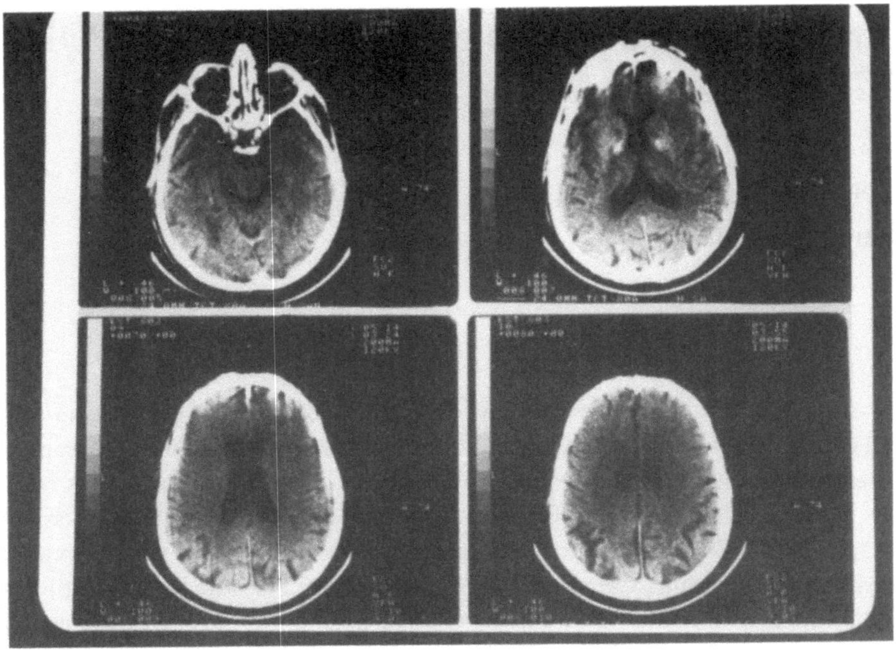

a

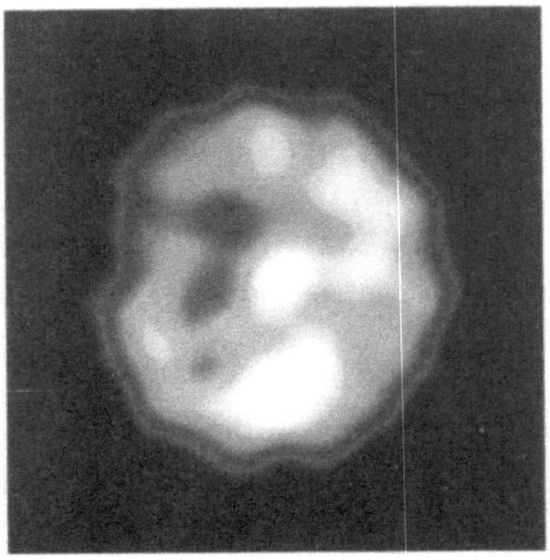

b

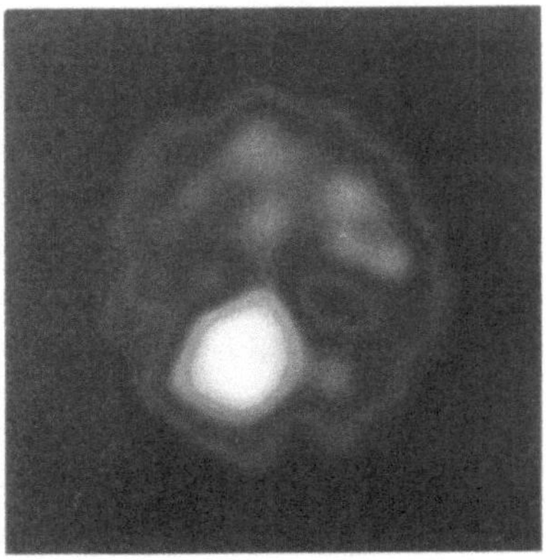

c

Fig. 1 Stroke of left cerebral hemisphere, investigated twelve hours after the onset.
a) CT scan shows roughly abnormalities (apart bilateral calcifications of the caudate nucleus); b) rCBF study (OM + 5.7 cm) shows decreased activity over the affected hemisphere, in the territory of the left middle cerebral artery; c) rCBF Study (OM + 0.3 cm) shows decreased activity over the right cerebellar hemisphere, related to crossed cerebellar diaschisis.

Patients with stroke

We studied 34 patients both in the early and late stage of brain infarction. In this kind of cerebral pathology, the ^{123}I HIPDM-SPECT technique allows:

a) early detection of damaged areas when CT scan is still negative (fig. 1);

b) functional delimitation of the ischemic area. In fact, and according to other

authors [4, 5, 6], the perfusion deficit visualized with Emission Tomography is often greater than the typical low-density area at CT scan;
c) detection of functional changes of rCBF at the site of lesion, such as luxury perfusion [7, 8];
d) evidentiation of functional remote effect such as crossed cerebellar diaschisis [9, 10, 11].

Prospective studies to evaluate recovery in the acute phase of stroke in respect to the degree of tissue perfusion deficit or to assess the ability of therapies to limit the

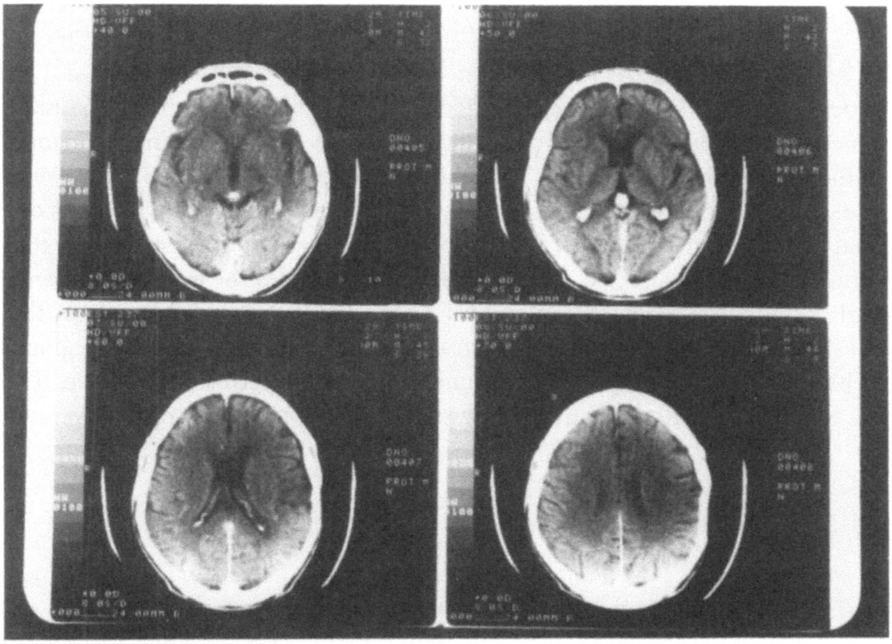

a

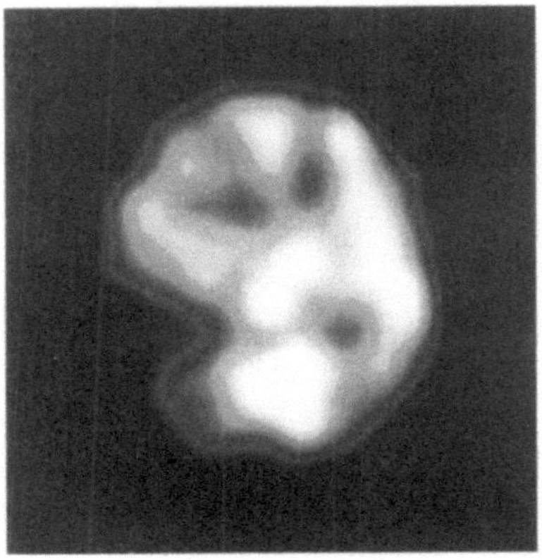

b

Fig. 2 Reversible ischemic attacks of left hemisphere:
a) CT scan is normal; b) rCBF study (OH + 5.7 cm) shows decreased activity over the left parieto-occipital region, probably relative to a state of critical perfusion.

extension of ischemic damage should be forthcoming. In fact the rCBF alone is only a limited aspect of cerebral energy values. In particular it doesn't reflect the complexities of pathophysiological changes in the acute post-infarct state. Only in conjunction with metabolic parameter rCBF will be of value to assess tissue viability (the ischemic penumbra).

However, ^{123}I HIPDM study may be an helpful method to detect the occurrence and to point the size of an ischemic injury more accurately than CT scan, and it may be potentially useful for the evaluation of therapeutical trials in the management of acute stroke.

Patients with R.I.A.

In 22 patients with Reversible Ischemic Attacks (RIAs), ^{123}I HIPDM-SPECT studies, in conjunction with other radioisotopic studies such as the assessment of regional cerebral blood volume (rCBF) by ^{99m}Tc labelled red blood cells [12, 13], may be of value to detect areas of critical perfusion [10, 14]. Patients presenting with RIAs due to internal carotid artery occlusion showed often a decrease in isotope activity, that is in perfusion, over the affected cerebral hemisphere besides the eventual presence of normal neurological examination and CT scan. (Fig. 2) Ischaemic events of this type may be the result of a state of critically reduced cerebral flow in regional cerebral blood volume in response to diminished cerebral perfusion pressure. The detection of areas of critical perfusion may suggest the opportunity of a preventive

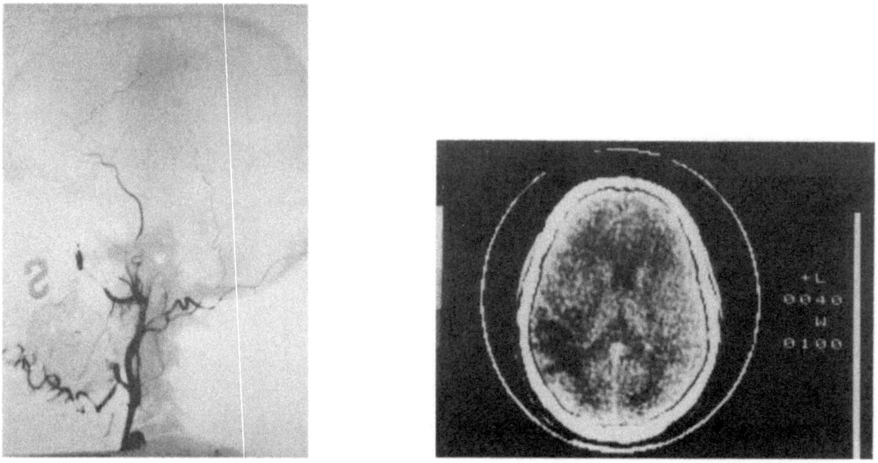

a b

Fig. 3 Minor stroke due to occlusion of left internal carotid artery (ICA) submitted to ECA-ICA by-pass surgery:
a) carotid angiography: occlusion of left ICA; b) CT scan shows an hypodense area in the left temporo-parietal region; c) rCBF study (OM + 3.3 cm) shows reduced activity in the territory of left ICA; d) Post-operative carotid angiography shows the patency of ECA-ICA by-pass; e) rCBF post-operative study (OM + 3.3 cm) shows increased activity in the territory of left ICA; f) rCBF study, 6 months after surgery (OM + 3.3 cm) shows that the activity in the territory of left ICA is now reduced back to pre-surgery levels.
Continued s. page 175

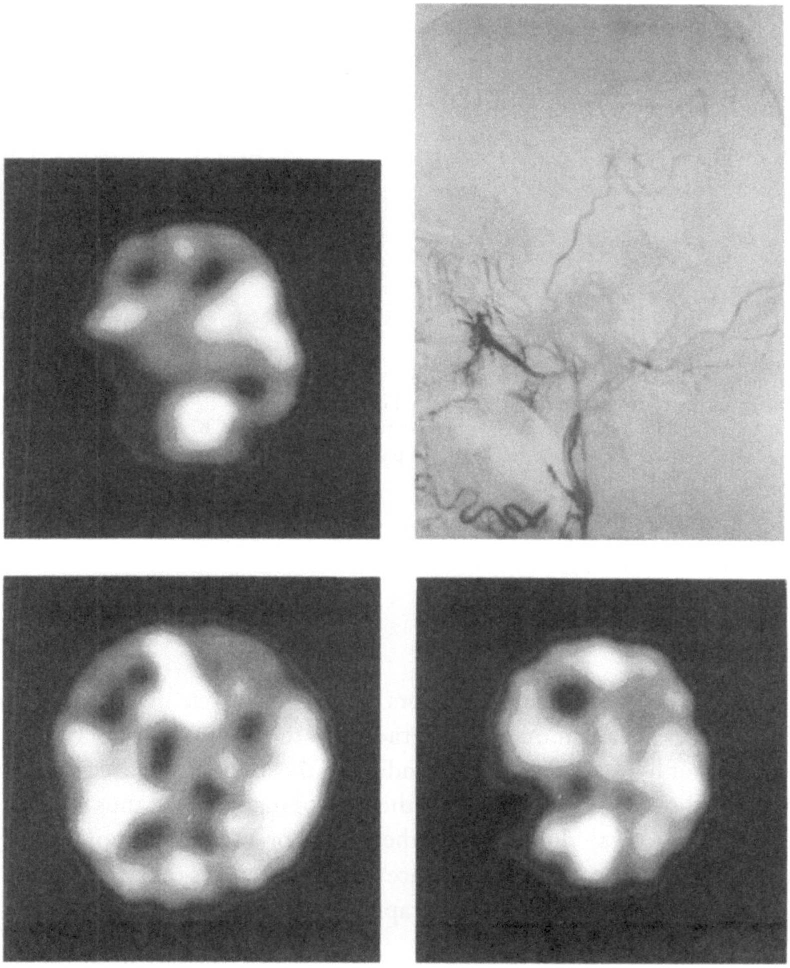

c d

e f

Fig. 3 *(Continued)*

surgical therapy with cerebral revascularization by anastomosis between external and internal carotid artery (EC-IC).

Patients with EC-IC by-pass

We evaluated rCBF in 16 patients submitted to EC-IC by-pass surgery. Before surgery, the perfusion study showed in all patients cortical areas of reduced ^{123}I HIPDM distribution in the affected hemisphere, in presence of normal or minimally impaired CT scan. Shortly after EC-IC by-pass and angiographic control of its patency, an increase of ^{123}I HIPDM uptake was detected in the same areas. Six months later, rCBF study was repeated, after angiographic control, showing mainly a decrease of activity with respect to the previous post-operative rCBF study. In respect to the pre-operative studies, rCBF was highly variable, appearing increased, decreased or unchanged. These findings tend to indicated that for any evaluation of

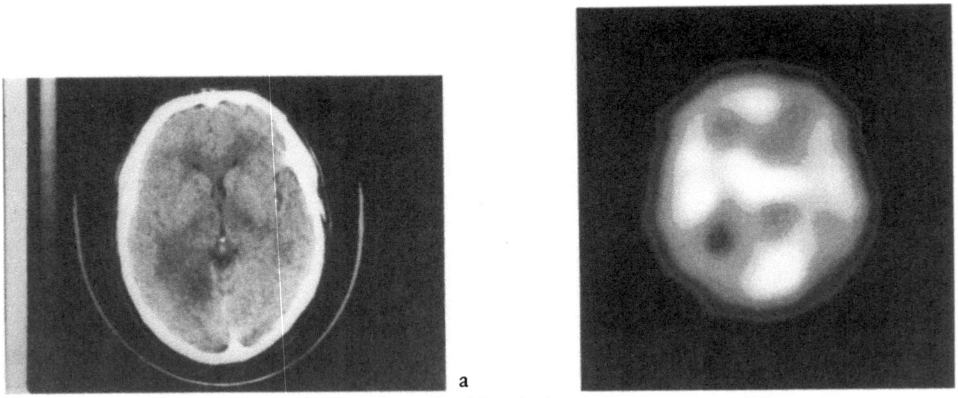

Fig. 4 Low grade astrocytoma in the left cerebral hemisphere:
a) CT scan shows an hypodense area in the left hemisphere; b) rCBF study (OM + 4.5 cm) shows a reduced activity area in the left temporo-parietal-occipital regions.

reperfusion after EC-IC by-pass, a direct assessment of rCBF is essential. By-pass patency per se is not an indicator of final reperfusion. (Fig. 3)

Cerebral tumours

We studied also few cases of brain tumors. In particular, we investigated atrocytomas to evaluate the localization and the grading of the tumor. The ^{123}I HIPDM study showed regions of hypoactivity corresponding to the low-density areas evidenced by CT scan but without a relationship with the type of malignancy, thus resulting of no help for the differential diagnosis of the grade of malignancy of astrocytoma. However, rCBF could be useful to evidence tissue alterations that are isodense at CT scan and to evaluate the efficacy of therapies. (Fig. 4)

Epilepsy

Four cases of epilepsy have been studied. Two patients were injected during the occurrence of generalized seizure type absence, induced by hyperventilation and recorded by EEG monitoring. ^{123}I HIPDM-SPECT studies didn't show asymmetry of activity of the tracer either interhemispheric either intrahemispheric.

In conclusion, SPECT studies with ^{123}I HIPDM are of clinical utility for the assessment and the haemodynamic physiopathological evaluation of neurological disorders, being thus complementary to CT scan. Being non invasive and only requiring accessible instrumentation, the method has the potential for becoming a routine clinical tool.

Up to date, main limitations of the method are the considerable planning required, the cost associated with the supply of ^{123}I and, finally, the difficulties to obtain an absolute quantitative measurement of rCBF.

References

[1] Kung, H. F., K. M. Tramposch, M. Blau: A new brain perfusion imaging agent: (^{123}I)HIPDM: N,N,N'-trimethyl-N'-(2-hydroxy-3-methyl-5-iodobenzyl) -1,3-propanediamine. J. Nucl. Med. **24** (1983) 66–72.

[2] Lucignani, G., F. Fazio, A. Nehlig et al.: Evaluation of (^{123}I) HIPDM as a potential tracer for the measurement of regional cerebral blood flow (abstract). In: Methods of cerebral blood flow and metabolism measurements in man. (Hartmann, A., Hoyer, S. eds.) Springer-Verlag, Berlin 1983 (in press).

[3] Fazio, F., G. I. Lenzi, P. Gerundini et al.: Tomographic assessment of regional cerebral perfusion using intravenous ^{123}I HIPDM and a rotating gamma camera. J. Comput. Assist. Tomogr. **8** (5) (1984) 911–924.

[4] Ell, P. J., I. Cullum, M. Donaghy et al.: Cerebral blood flow studies with ^{123}iodine-labelled amines. Lancet **1** (1983) 1348–52.

[5] Hill, T. C., P. L. Magistretti, B. L. Holman et al.: Assessment of regional cerebral blood flow (rCBF) in stroke using SPECT and N-isopropyl-(^{123}I)-p-iodoamphetamine (IMP). Stroke **15** (1984) 40–45.

[6] von Schulthess, G. K., E. Ketz, P. A. Schubiger et al.: Regional quantitative noninvasive assessment of cerebral perfusion and function with N-isopropyl-(^{123}I)p-iodoamphetamine. J. Nucl. Med. **26** (1985) 9–16.

[7] Lassen, N. A.: The luxury-perfusion syndrome and its possible relation to acute metabolic acidosis localised within the brain. Lancet ii (1966) 1113–5.

[8] Skyhoy Olsen T., B. Larsen, E. Beek Skriver et al.: Focal cerebral hyperemia in acute stroke. Stroke **12** (1981) 598–606.

[9] Baron, J. C., M. G. Bousser, D. Comar et al.: Crossed cerebellar diaschisis in human supratentorial brain infarction (abstract.) Ann. Neurol. **8** (1980) 128.

[10] Lenzi, G. L., R. S. J. Frackowiak, T. Jones: Cerebral oxygen metabolism and blood flow in human cerebral ischemic infarction. J. Cerebr. Blood. Flow. Metab. **2** (1981) 231–35.

[11] Meneghetti, G., S. Vorstrup, B. Mickey et al.: Crossed cerebellar diaschisis in ischemic stroke: a study of regional cerebral blood flow by ^{133}Xe inhalation and single photon emission computerized tomography. J. Cerebr. Blood. Flow. Metab. **4** (1984) 235–240.

[12] Kuhl, D. E., M. Reivich, A. Alavi et al.: Local cerebral blood volume determined by three-dimensional reconstruction of radionuclide scan data. Circulation Research **36** (1975) 610–619.

[13] Gibbs, J. M., R. J. S. Wise, K. L. Leenders et al.: Evaluation of cerebral perfusion reserve in patients with carotid-artery occlusion. Lancet i (1984) 310–314.

[14] Baron, J. C., M. G. Bousser, D. Comar et al.: Reversal of focal "misery-perfusion syndrome" by extra-intracranial arterial bypass in hemodynamic cerebral ischemia. Stroke **12** (1981) 454–459.

List of contributors

Auf, E., Abteilung für Neuronuklearmedizin, Neurologische Universitätsklinik, Wien, Austria
Askienazy, S., Hôpital St.-Anne, Paris, France

Baldwin, R. M., Medi + Physics, Richmond/CA, USA
Bekier, A., Institut für Nuklearmedizin, Kantonspital, St. Gallen, Switzerland
Biersack, H. J., Institut für klinische und experimentelle Nuklearmedizin der Universität, Bonn, FRG
Bischof-Delaloye, A., Centre Hospitalier Universitaire Vaudois, Div. Autonome des Médécine Nucleaire, Lausanne, Switzerland
Brücke, Th., Neurologische Universitätsklinik, Wien, Austria
de Bruïne, J. F., Department of Radiology, Academic Medical Center, Amsterdam, Netherlands
Bülau, P., Universitäts Nervenklinik/Epileptologie, Bonn, FRG
Buell, U., Abteilung Nuklearmedizin/Zentrum für Radiologie, RWTH, Aachen, FRG

Cesare, P., Instituto S. Raphaele, University of Milan, Dept. of Neuroscience, University of Rome
Creutzig, H., Abteilung Nuklearmedizin/Universitätskliniken GHS, Essen, FRG

Dal Bianco, P., Abteilung für Neuronuklearmedizin, Neurologische Universitätsklinik, Wien, Austria
Delaloye, B., Div. Autonome de Médécine Nucleaire, Centre Hospitalier Universitaire Vaudois, Lausanne, Switzerland
Del Maschio, A., Instituto S. Raphaele, University of Milan, Dept. of Neuroscience, University of Rome
Di Piero, V., Dept. of Nuclear Medicine, University of Milan, Italy

Ell, P. J., Institute of Nuclear Medicine, Middlesex Hospital Medical School, London, England
Einhäupl, K., Abteilung Nuklearmedizin, Radiologische Universitätsklinik, Klinikum Großhadern, München, FRG

Fazio, F., Dept. of Nuclear Medicine, University of Milan, Italy
Fischer, R., Abteilung Nuklearmedizin, Universitätsklinik, Freiburg, FRG
Fröscher, W., Abteilung Neurologie, Psychiatrisches Landeskrankenhaus Weißenau, Ravensburg-Weißenau, FRG

Gerundini, P., Instituto S. Raphaele, University of Milan, Dept. of Neuroscience, University of Rome, Italy
Goldenberg, G., Abteilung für Neuronuklearmedizin, Neurologische Universitätsklinik, Wien, Austria

Harrison, R. C., Amersham International plc, Buckinghamshire, England
Hill, T. C., Dept. of Radiology, Harvard Medical School, Boston, USA
Höll, K., Abteilung für Neuronuklearmedizin, Neurologische Universitätsklinik, Wien, Austria
Holman, B. L., Dept. of Radiology, Harvard Medical School, Boston, USA
Hundeshagen, H., Abteilung für Nuklearmedizin und spezielle Biophysik, Medizinische Hochschule, Hannover, FRG

de Jong, J. M. B. V., Dept. of Experimental Neurology, Academic Medical Center, Amsterdam, Netherlands

Klünenberg, H., Amersham Buchler GmbH, Braunschweig, FRG
Knapp, F. F., Nuclear Medicine Group, Health and Safty Research Division, Oak Ridge National Laboratory, Oak Ridge/Tennessee, USA
Knust, E. J., Institut für medizinische Strahlenphysik und Strahlenbiologie, Universitätsklinikum, Essen, FRG
Krappel, W., Abteilung Nuklearmedizin/Radiologische Universitätsklinik, Klinikum Großhadern, München, FRG

Lamb, J. F., Medi + Physics, Richmond/CA, USA
Lenzi, P. L., Instituto S. Raphaele, University of Milan, Dept. of Neuroscience, University of Rome, Italy
Lin, Tz-Hong, Medi + Physics, Richmond/Ca, USA

Machulla, H. J., Institut für medizinische Strahlenphysik und Strahlenbiologie, Universitätsklinikum, Essen, FRG
Meili, A., Abteilung für Nuklearmedizin, Kantonspital, St. Gallen, Switzerland
Meyer, G. J., Institut für Nuklearmedizin und spezielle Biophysik, Medizinische Hochschule, Hannover, FRG
Moore, S. C., Dept. of Radiology, Harvard Medical School, Boston, USA
Moretti, J. L., Hôpital Henry Mondor, Service de Médécine Nucleaire, Creteil, France
Mueller, S. P., Dept. of Radiology, Harvard Medical School, Boston, USA

Neirinckx, R. D., Amersham International plc, Buckinghamshire, England
Nowotnik, D. P., Amersham International plc, Buckinghamshire, England

Penin, H., Neurologische Universitätsklinik/Epileptologie, Bonn, FRG
Pfeiffer, G., Mallinckrodt-Diagnostica, Wien, Austria
Pickett, R. D., Amersham International plc, Buckinghamshire, England
Podreka, I., Abteilung für Neuronuklearmedizin, Neurologische Universitätsklinik, Wien, Austria

Raynaud, C., Service Frédéric Joliot, Hôpital d'Orsay, Orsay, France
Reichmann, K., Institut für klinische und experimentelle Nuklearmedizin der Universität, Bonn, FRG
von Royen, E. A., Dept. of Nuclear Medicine, Academic Medical Center, Amsterdam, Netherlands

Savi, A., Instituto S. Raphaele, University of Milan, Dept. of Neuroscience, University of Rome, Italy
Sergent, A., Clinical Neurosciences Dept., CHU H. Mondor, Creteil, France
Schmiedek, P., Neurochirurgische Universitätsklinik, Klinikum Großhadern, München, FRG
Schober, O., Institut für Nuklearmedizin und spezielle Biophysik, Medizinische Hochschule, Hannover, FRG
van der Schoot, J. B., Dept. of Nuclear Medicine, Academic Medical Center, Amsterdam, Netherlands
Schuemichen, C., Abteilung für Nuklearmedizin, Universitätsklinik, Freiburg, FRG
von Schulthess, G. K., Radiologische Universitätsklinik, Zürich, Switzerland
Srivastava, P. C., Nuclear Medicine Group, Oak Ridge National Laboratory, Oak Ridge/Tennessee, USA
Strauß, E., Abteilung für Nuklearmedizin, Universitätsklinik, Freiburg, FRG

Tardy, Clinical Neurosciences Dept. CHU H. Mondor, Creteil, France
Triulzi, F., Instituto S. Raphaele, University of Milan, Dept. of Neuroscience, University of Rome, Italy

Venema, H., Dept. of Radiology, Academic Medical Center, Amsterdam, Netherlands
Vyth, A., Dept. of Nuclear Medicine, Academic Medical Center, Amsterdam, Netherlands

Weder, B., Institut für Nuklearmedizin, Kantonspital, St. Gallen, Switzerland
Wimberger, D., Abteilung für Neuronuklearmedizin, Neurologische Universitätsklinik, Wien, Austria

Winkler, C., Institut für klinische und experimentelle Nuklearmedizin der Universität, Bonn, FRG
Wu, Jiann-Long Medi + Physics Richmond/CA, USA

Author's index

Subject index

Bei Fragen zur Produktsicherheit wenden Sie sich bitte an:
If you have any questions regarding product safety,
please contact:

Walter de Gruyter GmbH
Genthiner Straße 13
10785 Berlin
productsafety@degruyterbrill.com